CW00520199

The Offshore Grand Prix
There's No Turning Back

The Offshore Grand Prix
There's No Turning Back

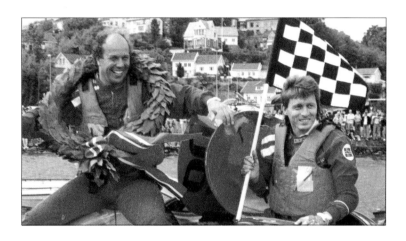

Step into the world of the UIM Offshore Grand Prix

with your hosts, The Ugland Team

By Jill Berg

Produced & Published by Cross Publishing, Newport, Isle of Wight, England

ISBN 1 873295 45 6

Table of Contents

In Gratitude To...

T he Ugland Team and the author would like to take this opportunity to thank all those people who have supported the writing of this book.

First thanks must go to the photographers who donated their priceless photos. Several names stand out. The majority of the photos came from the eagle eyes of Leo Kennedy and Derrick Lloyd. Special shots were donated by Chris Davies and Glen Philip Hagen. Other photography was donated directly from the teams: *KR Racing Team, Achilli Motors Racing Team, Ferretti Racing Team, Antonio Gioffredi* and the *Victory Team*. Photography was also donated by Dr. Matt Houghton of the Mark Lavin Memorial Safety Foundation.

Thanks must also go to Mauro Ravenna and his staff at SPES and Gianfranco Zanoni for helping locate the teams when we were doing research on each of the competitors. Derrick and Jane Lloyd were also very helpful in "filling in the rough spots" on the text. The notes he kept while doing commentary for Dubai Television proved incredibly valuable. Norman Gentry's analysis of the chapter on technology helped clarify a lot of the text in that chapter as well.

Finally, the team would like to thank Svein Backe and the Norwegian Powerboat Association for all their support over the years. The NPA was every bit responsible for nurturing and encouraging the team to grow.

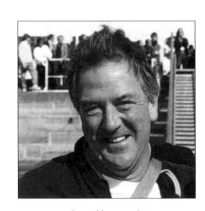

Leo Kennedy
Contributing Photographer.

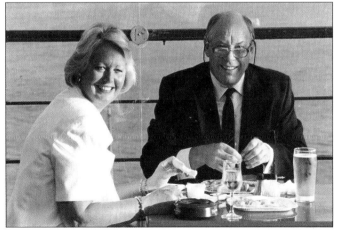

Jane and Derrick Lloyd
Contributing Photographer and Copy Consultant.

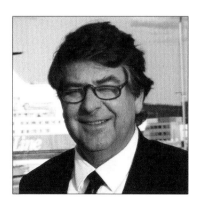

Svein Backe
President of the Norwegian
Powerboat Association.

The Offshore Grand Prix
There's No Turning Back

by Jill Berg

Introduction

It would be impossible to tell the story of The Offshore Grand Prix, the premiere circuit of offshore powerboat racing, without introducing you to the people. From race to race, season after season, it's the racers whose names cover the international headlines that make offshore racing interesting. How can you enjoy a sport without knowing what the competitors stand to loose, what they went through to get where they are, and who they are as people? To truly appreciate a sport we need some connection to it. Knowing the people immersed in competition, seeing their struggles, feeling their pains and enjoying their triumphs makes following a sport worthwhile.

And so, when undertaking this book, I chose to look at the sport through The Ugland Racing Team from Norway.

I chose The Ugland Team for several reasons. First of all, I had worked directly for the team as their public relations person in 1993 and had witnessed the experiences they shared in offshore racing first hand. Secondly, I chose to write about The Ugland Team because they are well rounded in the sport. Both the driver, Andreas Ove Ugland, and the throttleman, Jann Hillestad, competed in smaller classes, traveling up through the ranks from Class III and Class II, before racing in Class I. Therefore they have the knowledge necessary to compare the differences in racing between the three classes. Thirdly, although Andreas and Jann are very much alike, they are also two very distinct and interesting personalities. They feel the sport from two different perspectives, but together they're one of the best liked, and most competitive teams on the circuit. And finally, I chose to write about The Ugland Team because they represent the best in offshore. They are 100% professional at all times while remaining easy-going and likeable. They enjoy sharing their love of racing with others, which makes it possible for me to share their story with you.

This book follows The Ugland Team along their quest for a World Championship. Throughout your reading I'll strive to familiarize you with the terms used in the sport, as well as the sport itself, the competition, the safety guidelines and the technology as well as some of the light-hearted moments teams enjoy as they travel around the world on the Grand Prix circuit.

In the end you'll learn about offshore racing while getting to know some of the people involved. Short of actually being in a race, I hope this book is the next best thing.

Jill Berg

Chapter 1
The Ugland Offshore Race Team

Andreas Ugland is streaking along the ocean at over 100 miles an hour. Adrenaline pumps through his body as his digital speedometer climbs higher and higher. He searches the horizon for the first turn buoy, his navigational equipment clicking away on his dashboard. He's seen better days for racing. Today's seas are irregular, the waves choppy, with rollers coming in as high as seven feet, their troughs falling just as deep. Andreas must read the waves carefully...must stay on top of their every shifting move. If he misses the span between waves, his boat can drop 14 feet straight down.

Over and over Andreas feels his body being slammed back and forth in his seat. A five point harness system protects and contains him, pulling against his shoulders, pinching and strapping him in place. The whites of his knuckles strain against his racing gloves as he tightens his grip on the steering wheel.

Seated directly behind Andreas, his throttleman Jann Hillestad controls the speed, accelerating the boat to 110, 120...over 130 miles per hour. Using his entire body, he switches on the two engine's turbos with his left foot and adjusts the trim tabs with his fingertips, all while pushing down on the throttles. Both men realize their life is in each other's hands...one misguided turn from Andreas, one miscalculation from Jann, and their 46 foot catamaran could spin out, hook or plow right under the waves.

The two work together in beautiful synchronization. Andreas steers, navigating, and calculating their competitions progress. Jann works the throttles, trims the boat and sets the turbos, blasting their boat towards victory. Andreas and Jann are Offshore Grand Prix racers. Together they make up one of the best racing teams in the world.

A host of twenty seven other boats race alongside them, heading into the first turn. With the sound of over 50,000 horsepower's worth of engines screaming in their ears, a tight knot forms in Andreas' throat, and Jann feels a gaping hole in the pit of his stomach. Turn One lies directly in front of them, a crowd of spectator boats are anchored off to their port side, forming an unofficial chute for the turn. It is impossible for so many boats to take this turn at once! Someone will have to back off. Andreas and Jann are out front this race. They've pushed hard to get where they are and are determined not to back down.

A helicopter suddenly looms above them, a cameraman hanging from an open door trying to take their picture. The turbulence from the chopper sends the water below them swirling into a sea of whirlpools. An invisible suction from the helicopter pulls up at the bow of their catamaran, dangerously lifting the boat out of the water.

The first turn is one of the most dangerous moments in an Offshore Grand Prix, but for the many competitors like Andreas and Jann, it is the most exciting. With twenty eight boats competing in each event in 1993, it is a wonder more accidents didn't occur. Jann and Andreas realize the odds are that it will happen. Both pray it won't be them.

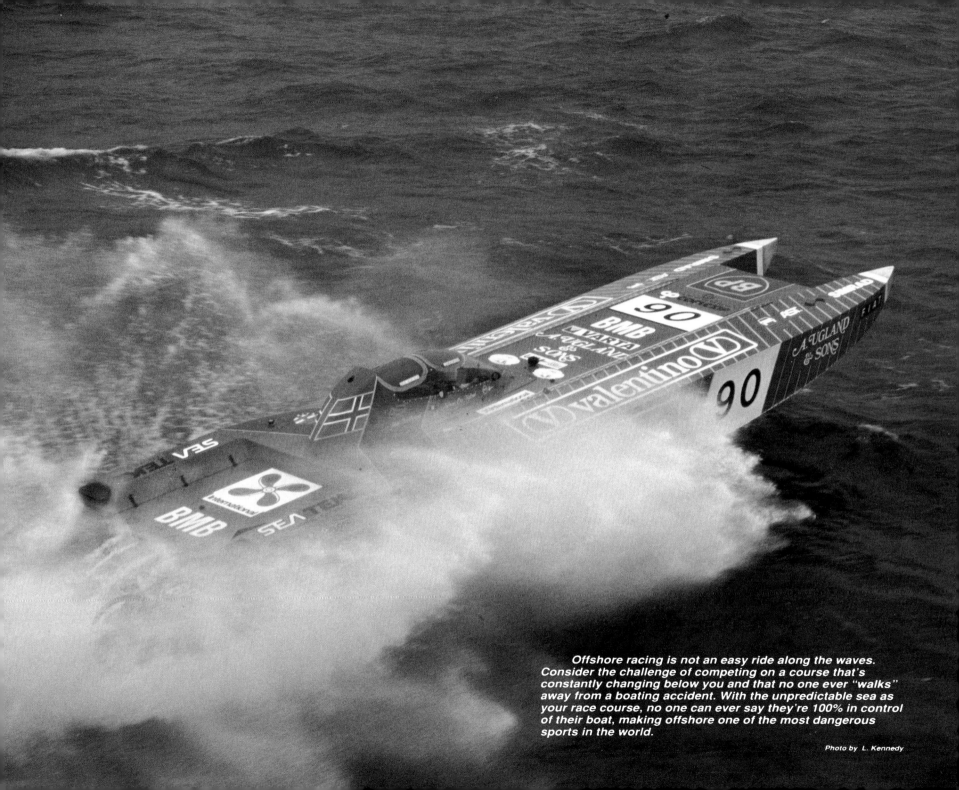

Offshore racing is not an easy ride along the waves. Consider the challenge of competing on a course that's constantly changing below you and that no one ever "walks" away from a boating accident. With the unpredictable sea as your race course, no one can ever say they're 100% in control of their boat, making offshore one of the most dangerous sports in the world.

Photo by L. Kennedy

Andreas Ove Ugland

Andreas Ove Ugland must have had boat racing genes in him on the day he was born. Hailing from the tiny town of Grimstad on the southern coast of Norway, Andreas and his two brothers, Johan and Knut, began powerboating with their parents along the fjords and seas near their home. Their father, Andreas K. Ugland, owner of an international shipping company, spent much of his time on business trips, leaving the three boys with their mother in Grimstad. As can be expected, the high spirited Ugland boys couldn't resist the opportunity for an occasional boat ride, a decision which usually got them into trouble, if not with their mother, then with the local kystvakt, the Norwegian coast guard.

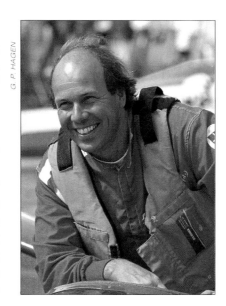

"The kystvakt knew my brothers and I very well," Andreas recalls fondly. "I think they just waited outside the fjords near our dock for one of us to come racing out. I'm sure they even pulled over my father thinking they'd caught one of us boys."

Of the three Ugland boys, Andreas, the middle son, was most avid in boating, ultimately convincing his grandfather, a retired ship builder, to help him build his first boat, an 8 foot, 6 horsepower monohull capable of reaching 18 miles an hour. The boat was a dream come true for young Andreas, and he was all the prouder of the small craft having experienced first hand the work painstakingly put into her hull.

It wasn't long, however, before Andreas dreamt of speeds beyond his boat's capabilities. Andreas attempted to join the Norwegian Powerboat Association (NPA), the national authority to the Union of Internationale Motonautique (UIM).

Unfortunately, the minimum age for NPA racing was 16, leaving Andreas to spend summer after summer watching the older boys compete without him.

"I couldn't wait for my first official race," Andreas explains. "My brother Johan was two years older than I, and even now I recall the torture of watching him compete when I was still too young. There was nothing I wanted more than to race, and especially race well enough to beat my brother. So, as soon as I could manage, I lied a year on my age and started racing when I was fifteen."

Once getting his name on the line-up, Andreas threw his passions into the NPA's circuit racing program. There, in a small 15 foot fiberglass catamaran built for one, he competed on a mile long course, taking him 20-25 laps each race.

While Andreas' passion for racing grew, so did he. As he matured Andreas married and became involved in the family business. Johan's interests ultimately turned towards other sports, while his younger brother Knut favored hunting and fishing to racing. This left Andreas the sole Ugland on the racing program.

Andreas did well in circuit racing, winning races and breaking the Nordic Speed Record in Class S-D with a speed of 101 kph. Andreas finally had to bow out of regular competition when he moved to the United States to earn both a Bachelor and Masters degree in Economics, Finance and International Trade from New York University.

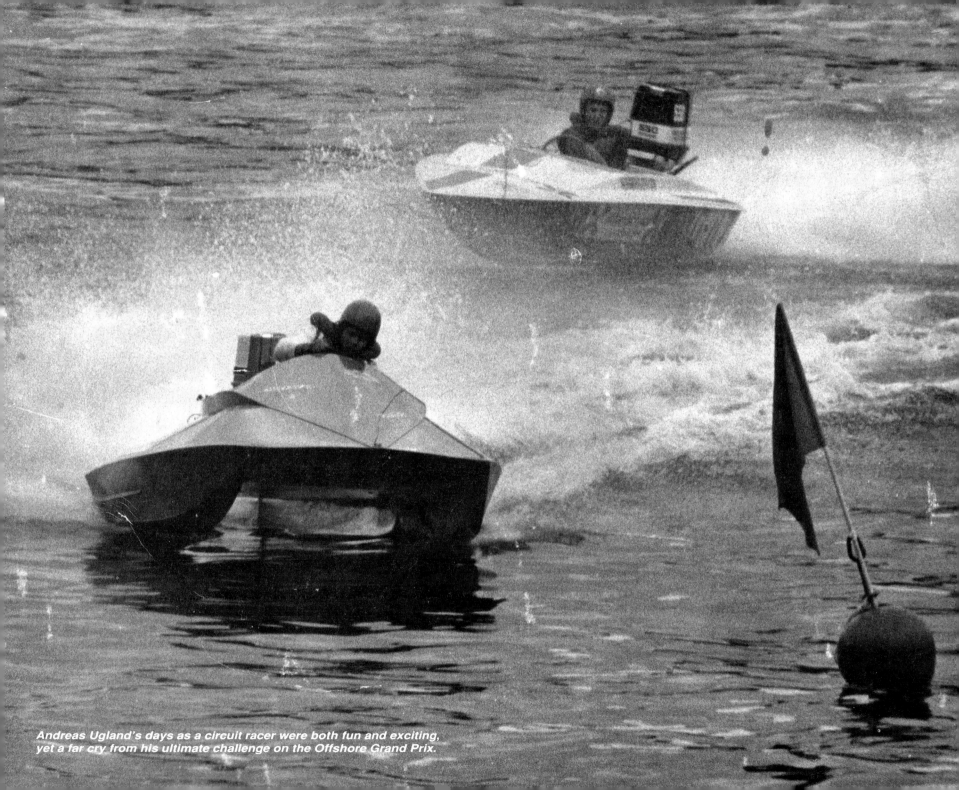

Andreas Ugland's days as a circuit racer were both fun and exciting, yet a far cry from his ultimate challenge on the Offshore Grand Prix.

Jann Hillestad

Jann Hillestad's interest in boat racing stems from his insatiable interest in technology, engineering, physics, and his love for sports others find dangerous.

Born in Lillehammer, Norway, Jann and his twin brother Svein grew up exposed to a world where sports and technology were advancing daily. Jann's intrigue into science lead to a career in engineering and computer technology, as well as serving on the board of Svein's international trading and electronic ship charting businesses. Yet, Jann's thrill seeking nature couldn't hold him back from competing in all manners of skiing, hang gliding and powerboating. Not only did Jann want to ski more efficiently, set hang gliding records and see his powerboat running faster, but he also wanted to understand how the physics and engineering designs served to make this happen.

It was this love of technology that lead Jann to building race boats for other people before ever racing himself. Learning the practical craft of boat building from his grandfather, Jann was fascinated with how the technology and design of boat building could take an average hull and turn it into the best on the circuit. His understanding of the laws of physics taught him how to work

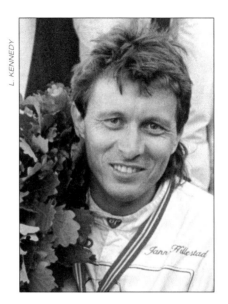

with nature to become not only a winning boat builder, but an ideal throttleman.

"Boat racing today is very different from when I first started," Jann reflects. "The technology was pretty basic then, but now it takes a very educated or mechanically minded person to sort out the details of a professional race boat. It's this ever changing technology that has kept my keen interest all these years."

Actively racing powerboats since 1973, Jann first became involved in the NPA's circuit racing program. One of the best circuit racers in the world, Jann moved through the different classes before ending his circuit racing career four years later as the winner of "6 Hour Paris Grand Prix" Formula 1 Class in 1977.

"Circuit racing is very different from offshore," Jann explains. "The boats carry only one driver, and I raced mine while lying on my stomach. I had fun, but after winning the 6 Hour Paris Grand Prix I was ready for something different."

Jann's rapid climb to the top of circuit boat racing made him yearn for new challenges. He would soon find them in a different form of boat racing, side by side with his friend and one time competitor Andreas Ugland.

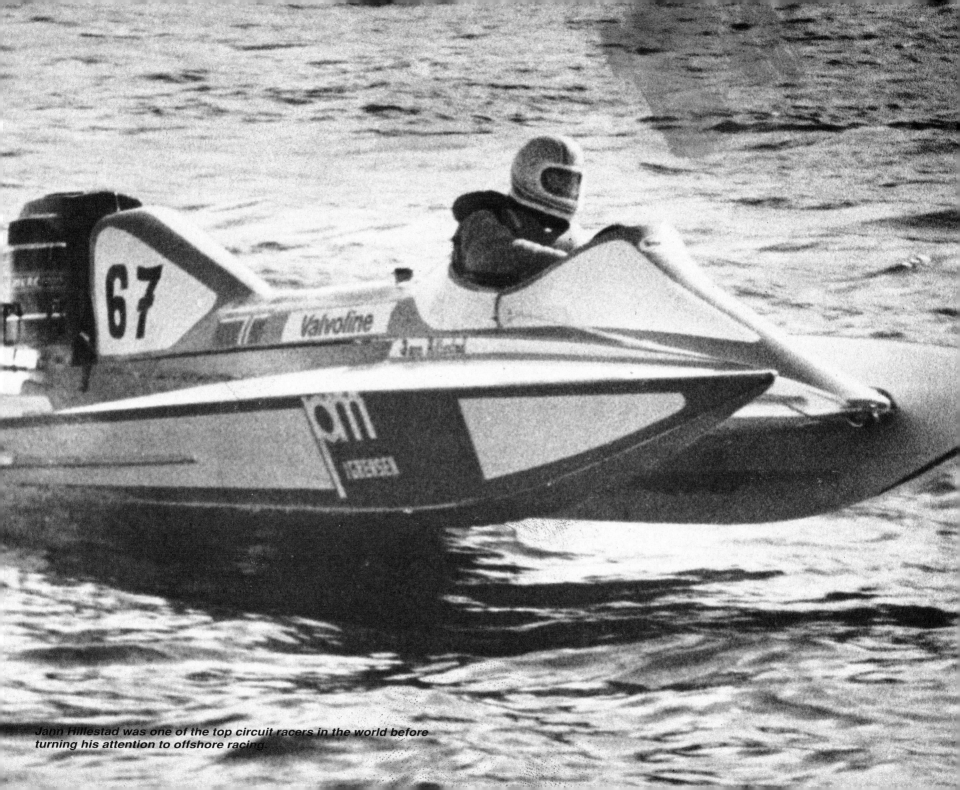

Jann Hillestad was one of the top circuit racers in the world before turning his attention to offshore racing.

Teaming Up

In the summer of 1988 Andreas met with Jann at a small restaurant in Ibiza for a conversation that would change their lives forever.

"I can remember our conversation as if it were yesterday," Jann reflects. "Andreas looked at me very seriously and said: "Jann, I feel we can be a very good team in offshore. Let's start out in Class III, then move up to Class II, and keep going and not give up before we are among the best in Class I." When Andreas asked me to be his throttleman, I took great consideration in the fact that Andreas is a man who always realizes the goals he makes for himself. I knew he had the determination to win, and that was all I needed to know to agree to his plans."

Racing together in Norway, Andreas and Jann soon earned reputations as serious competitors in Offshore Class III, the smallest UIM offshore class which provides professionally organized events for 19-20 foot, 4-liter stock boats built by such companies as Argo, Cougar and Skater. Racing in Class III the team competed in an about 8-10 races per year, competing against an average of fifteen other boats per event. The team ran in Class III for three years winning events throughout Norway and Europe in their

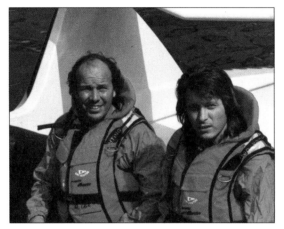

Andreas Ugland - Driver
Jann Hillestad - Throttleman

Frank Shorter Sportswear sponsored boat, before moving on to the next UIM Class, Class II.

UIM Class II is considered by many to be the training ground for the critically acclaimed UIM Class I. With their move into Class II, offshore racing became much more expensive for the Ugland duo, with The Ugland Group, Andreas' family's shipping company, ultimately becoming title sponsors. Racing in Class II, where hulls varied in length from 25 to 39 feet with 8 liter, 1,500 h.s.p engines, the Ugland Team became exposed to more international competition, a more extensive race schedule, and an increased number of international events as well as world-wide media coverage. Suddenly the two Norwegians were racing with the big boys.

Of the field, the Ugland duo's greatest rivals were Italy's Norberto Ferretti, famous for his fire-ball temper and aggressiveness on the course, Argentina's national hero Daniel Scioli and Italy's Andrea Bonomi, son of Carlo Bonomi, the builder of Ugland's Seatek diesel engines.

"Once in Class II Jann and I learned to work less as individuals and more as a team," Andreas explains. "Competing in larger boats against racers whose goals were to run Class I

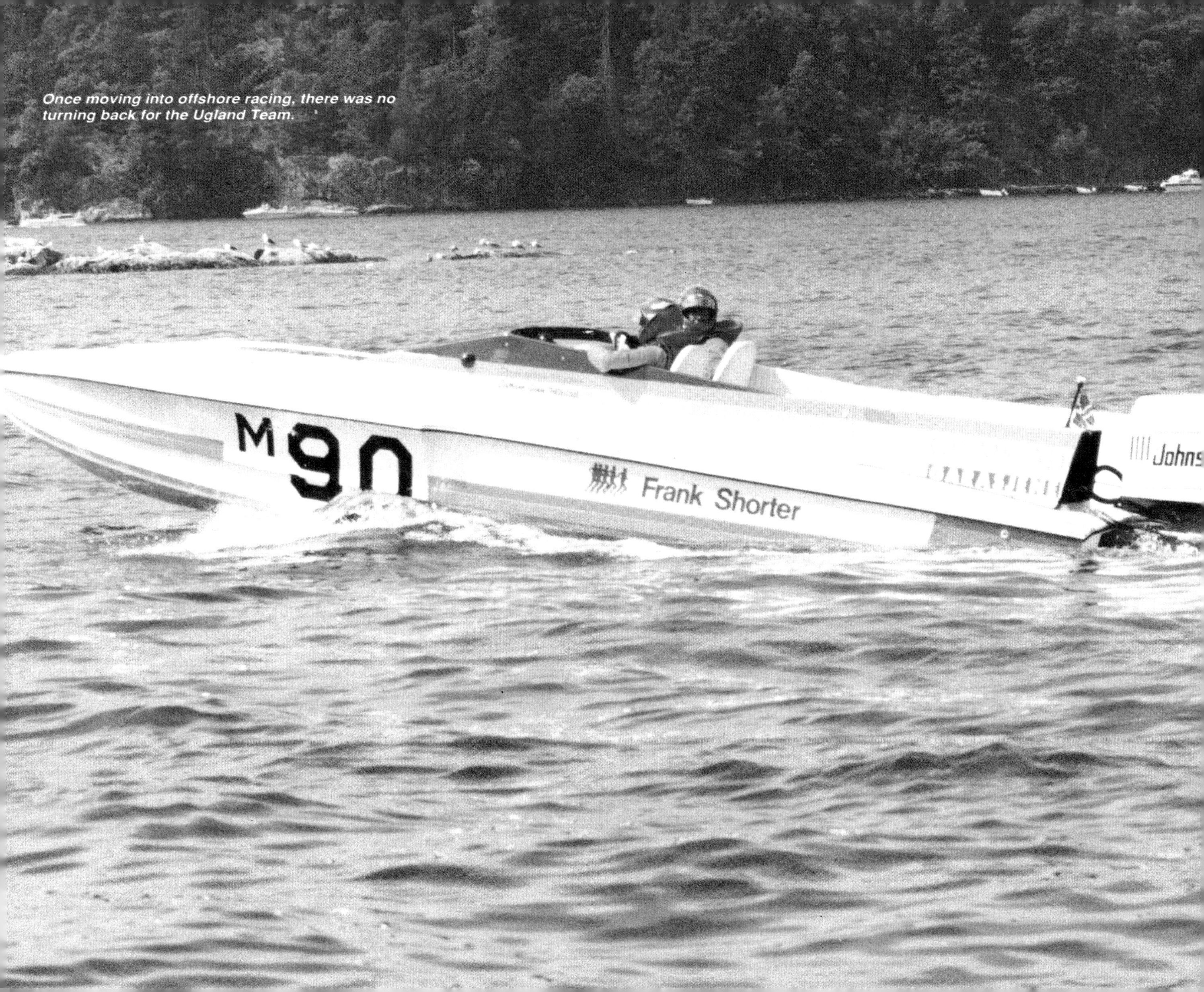

Once moving into offshore racing, there was no turning back for the Ugland Team.

made us run faster. Once speeds start hitting 100 m.p.h. you have to rely on the split second coordination between the driver and throttleman. That can only be developed over repeated competition together. Class II enabled Jann and I to find ourselves as a team."

Growing together as racers in Class II, the Ugland Team recognized their potential as winning competitors, witnessing their strengths and correcting any weaknesses.

"Andreas and I both grew so much in Class II," Jann explains. "His ability to feel the movements of the boat through the steering wheel is impressive. So many times I've seen the boat almost spin out in a turn, but Andreas would feel it exactly at the right moment and take whatever precautions necessary to prevent it. As I saw him do this over and over I learned to trust him, and now I almost take this talent of his for granted. I just expect him to keep us safe. Yet I can still recall how amazed I was, years ago, watching him do that the first few times."

Racing Class II in their Buzzi monohull, *The Ugland Group,* the duo was the only team to represent Norway, an honor both men took equal pride in. Racing Class II from 1987 until 1990, Andreas and Jann brought home 10 checkered flags, winning the hotly contested Class II European Championship of 1990.

The Ugland Team's successes in Class III and Class II earned them the ability to attract much needed sponsors, sponsorship they'd need to help absorb the expenses associated with competing on the international Class I circuit.

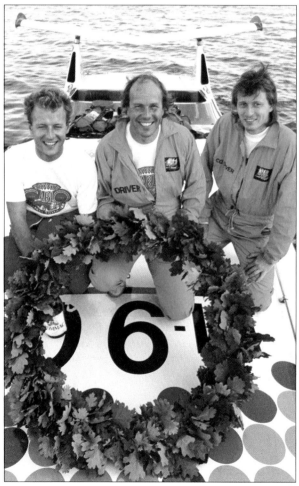

Luciano Togni served as navigator on The Ugland Group, helping Andreas and Jann win the 1990 European Championship in Class II.

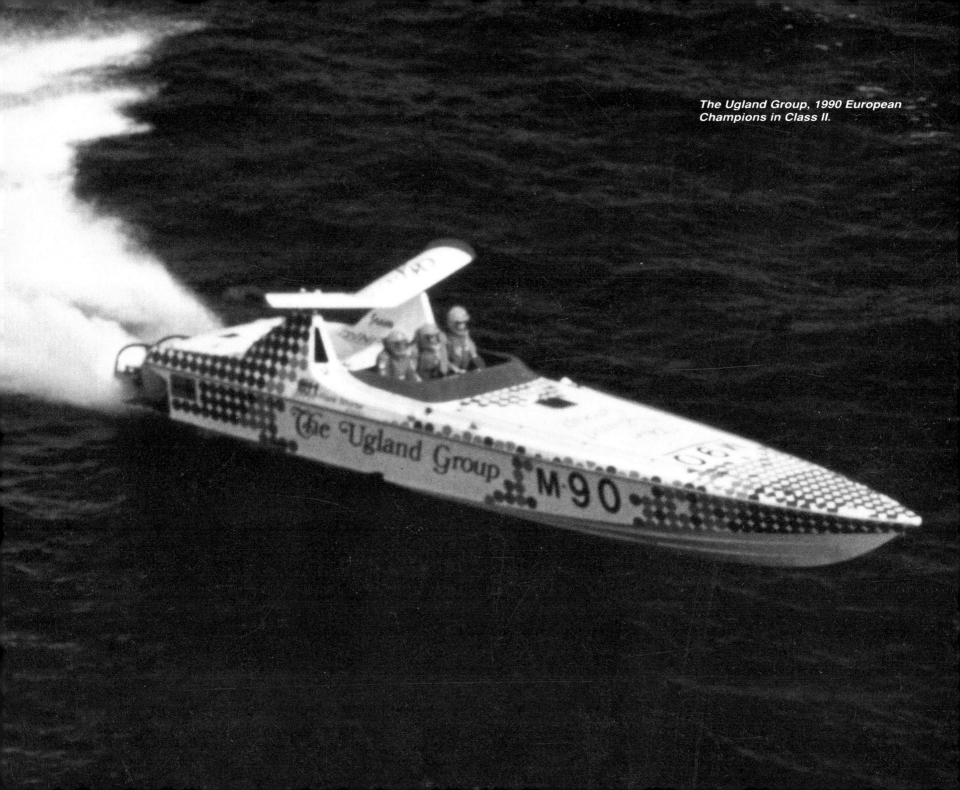

The Ugland Group, 1990 European Champions in Class II.

Chapter 2
From European Circuit to The Grand Prix

When Andreas Ugland and Jann Hillestad began racing Class I in 1991, they entered the class at a time of extreme change. Only the year before, at the 1990 World Championships in October, reigning World Champion Stefano Casiraghi, husband of Princess Caroline of Monaco, died defending his title. Suddenly the focus on the world was on Class I offshore racing.

With Casiraghi's death came new safety rules. Of the thirty or so boats racing at the time, all but a handful incorporated canopies, a clear plexiglass bubble covering the opening over the cockpit. Canopies were relatively new to offshore racing in 1990, but in 1991 safety rules were initiated making them mandatory, changing the appearance and costs of Class I dramatically. The typical offshore race boat no longer resembled hulls seen in boat yards and marinas around the world...they now looked like and became as costly as water-bound rocket ships.

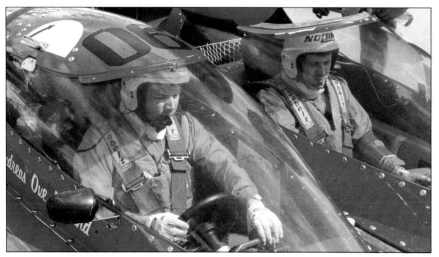

L. KENNEDY

The Fiat Uno

The Ugland Team entered Class I with a serious focus on safety equipment and hull design. After analyzing the locations of the various race sites they'd compete at, Andreas chose to commission a new 46 foot Buzzi monohull, complete with three 830 h.s.p. Seatek diesel engines, side-by-side split canopy cockpits, a five-point harness restraint system, underwater breathing apparatus and strengthened bulkhead.

Sponsored by Fiat Corporation and others, Ugland's *Fiat Uno*, was a true crowd pleaser, her bright red hull featuring an aerodynamic wing over the engine compartments, creating additional lift and stability to raise the 8-ton boat up and over the waves.

One of the few monohulls on the 1991 European circuit, the *Fiat Uno* was a gamble. Built for strength and stamina in rough water, monohulls are the perfect choice for open water racing, made to slice right through a wave. *Fiat Uno's* competition, however, came mostly from catamarans, boats whose hulls consist of two sponsons connected above the water line by a deck, the space underneath of which operates as a wind tunnel, lifting the entire boat to ride on top of waves. In rough water races *Fiat Uno's* winged monohull would have an advantage. In calm water, however, the lighter catamarans would be all but unstoppable. Because Andreas intended to compete on the European circuit as well as several long distance endurance races a monohull was determined to be the better choice for The Ugland Team's long term goals.

Canopies, such as those on Fiat Uno, became mandatory for Class I in 1991.

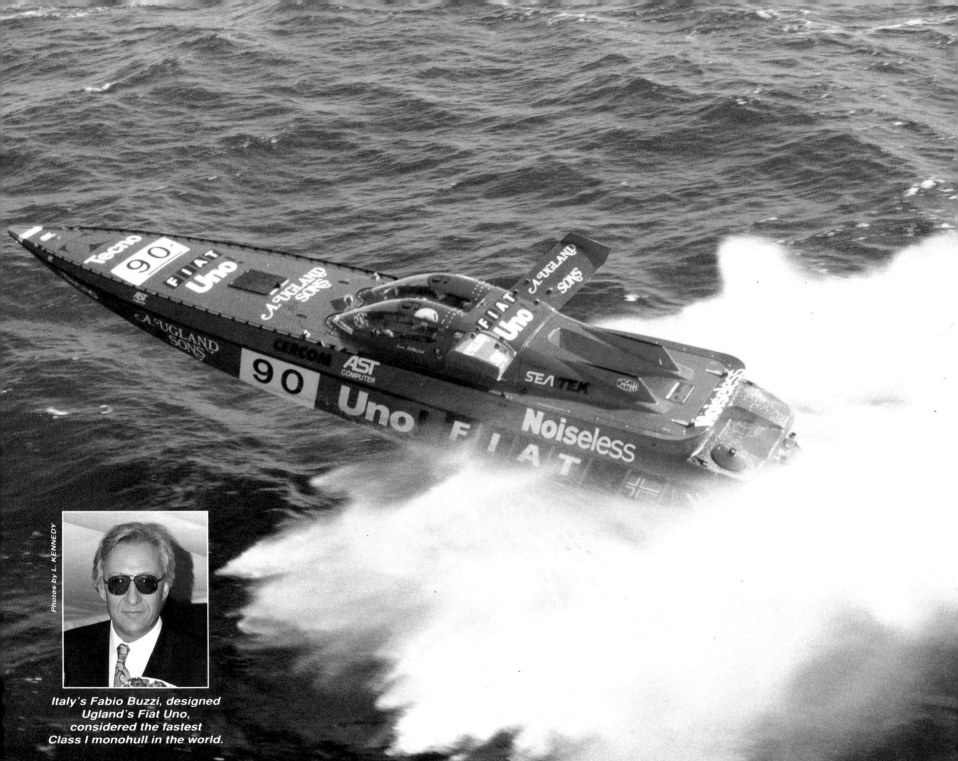

Photos by L. KENNEDY

Italy's Fabio Buzzi, designed Ugland's Fiat Uno, considered the fastest Class I monohull in the world.

The Crew

Backing up Andreas' and Jann's efforts in 1991 was the support crew that had been with them throughout their Class II racing; crew chief Gianfranco Zanoni, mechanic Svein Mykelbust, truck driver Johannes Aagre and team manager Leo Kennedy.

Gianfranco, an Italian, is a direct employee of Fabio Buzzi's FB Design, where he oversaw the construction of *Fiat Uno*. As crew chief, Gianfranco coordinates the mechanics from Italy and Norway and all technical aspects of the boat.

Svein and Johannes, both from Norway, have supported Andreas' racing as far back as his circuit racing days.

Johannes grew up near Andreas and has been his close friend for over 30 years. Svein handled Andreas' private boating concerns in Norway, working for him full time.

Team manager Leo Kennedy, a retired ship broker, is an English gentleman with a wealth of business contacts and a sharp eye behind a camera. As team manager, Leo's duties take him from sponsor board meetings and team photography to co-driving the team's motorhome with Johannes when the team competes in endurance races.

Together, Ugland's crew meshed into a professional team, one that worked well together during the tense, highly stressed racing season. While other teams may have had larger crews, the crew on *Fiat Uno* was every bit as effective.

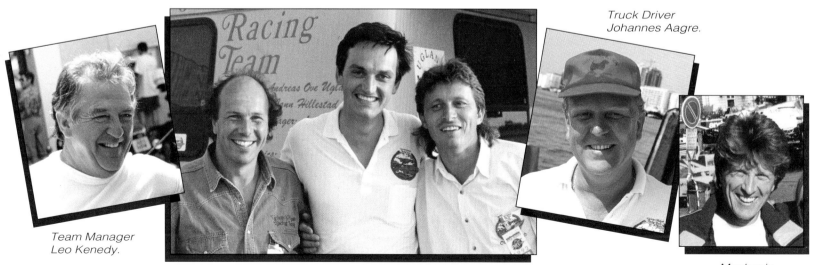

Truck Driver Johannes Aagre.

Team Manager Leo Kenedy.

Andreas Ugland, Crew Chief Gianfranco Zanoni, and Jann Hillestad.

Mechanic Svein Myklebust.

The Field on The European Circuit

Of the thirty teams in Class I in 1991, only a handful of the racers were from countries outside Italy. Competing on the 1991 European roster were Finland's J.P. Mattilla, Swiss racer Sandro Gianella, France's Bernard Coustenoble and Pascal Villanova, as well as Britian's Richard Carr and two-time World Champion Steve Curtis. Andreas and Jann were the only team to represent Norway.

"At first we felt somewhat isolated," Jann recalls, "however, our association with Fabio Buzzi opened a lot of doors for us. Once our competitors saw we were committed enough to work with someone of Buzzi's reputation, they took us seriously."

The competition in Class I had already heard of the Ugland Team, the reigning World Champions in Class II, as well as their fierce rivalry between fellow Class II racer Norberto Ferretti from Italy.

Unlike Ugland, Ferretti chose to compete in Class I in a catamaran. Weighing only 4,000 kg in full racing trim, the design of Ferretti's *Iceberg* was one of the most technologically advanced raceboats appearing in 1991.

Also running new boats was Carr's *Lamborghini Leisure*, a Lamborghini powered Cougar catamaran. Italy's Marco Capoterri also chose the British Cougar boat for his new *Sireg*, but opted for Seatek diesels. Domenico Achilli's new Stain catamaran was another beauty, aptly named *Achilli Motors* after his Italian luxury car franchise.

Finland's J.P. Mattila re-flagged his *Notareal* catamaran with new sponsor, *FinnScrew,* hoping to bring in more reliable finishes against the competitive Spelta and Polli families of Italy. Angelo

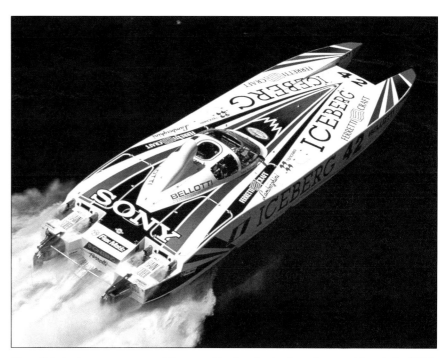

Ferretti's Iceberg was one of the most technologically advanced boats in 1991.

Spelta brought his two boat Nooxy Team, and with throttleman Maurizio Ambrogetti registered under *Fresh & Clean* sponsorship. His son, Damiano, registered his own entry, *GP Pedrini-Dalle Carbonare*, racing alongside throttleman Alissandro Zocchi.

Patriarch of the Polli's 3 boat Rainbow Team, Edoardo Polli chose to run his 4 engine *SDA*, an extremely quick but unreliable Birkitt catamaran. Nephew Vincenzo Polli ran with Steve Curtis in *Bagutta*, a new streamlined Cougar powered by Lamborghini, and Leonardo Polli took over the third Polli boat, *Unipol*.

Although an average of 30 boats would compete in each of the ten events on the 1991 circuit, these teams lead the field the majority of the races.

The 1991 European Championship Season

A brief look at the 1991 European Circuit - the year before the Grand Prix began - sheds some light on the situations that led to the Grand Prix. The schedule in 1991 did not cover all of Europe, instead concentrating on three races in France, two in Great Britain and six in Italy. These races were, on the whole, well run events carried out by individual race promoters from the local area, with coordination of their activities organized by the UIM Offshore Committee and Class I promoter Mauro Ravenna. Ravenna's talents, however, were focused on the World Championship finals held in Trieste, Italy that year.

The World Championship title was given to the winner accumulating the most points at the final three World Championship heats. In order to qualify for the World Championship competition, each team had only to compete in five regular season events. That meant races at the end of the season could fall victim to lower turnouts as teams high enough in the rankings chose to send their boats in for repairs or chose to skip races to save money. Race sites could never predict competitor turn-out. As many as thirty Class I race teams could line up for the start, or as few as fourteen. This unpredictability made it hard for sites to secure race site sponsorship, resulting in last minute race cancellations and questions on race quality as local organizers searched for ways to save money.

There was also a strong difference between the level of boats racing in Class I. With the best media coverage of the three offshore classes, fully sponsored teams and those needing sponsors all attempted to run Class I. Unfortunately, the lesser financed teams could not run competitively with teams carrying stronger backing and thus better equipment. Any given start in 1991 would illustrate that there were two fields in Class I. The premier boats, such as the Rainbow Team, the Spelta's, *Iceberg* and *Fiat Uno*, and an almost "sub" class within Class I. These teams couldn't make the start with the same speed as the leading boats. It seemed as if many teams were better equipped to run Class II and be leaders there instead of running Class I. This doubled the "packs" that the boats often run in, and also doubled the amount of safety coverage needed.

Class I was growing. And as with most growth comes growing pains. But in a sport where speed is the essence, the changes couldn't come fast enough.

A new venue was needed. Race sites throughout Europe. Tighter control of the level of competition. Guaranteed races. Better safety control. Stronger leadership. Questions were raised, and in typical fashion, the UIM was there to provide the answer.

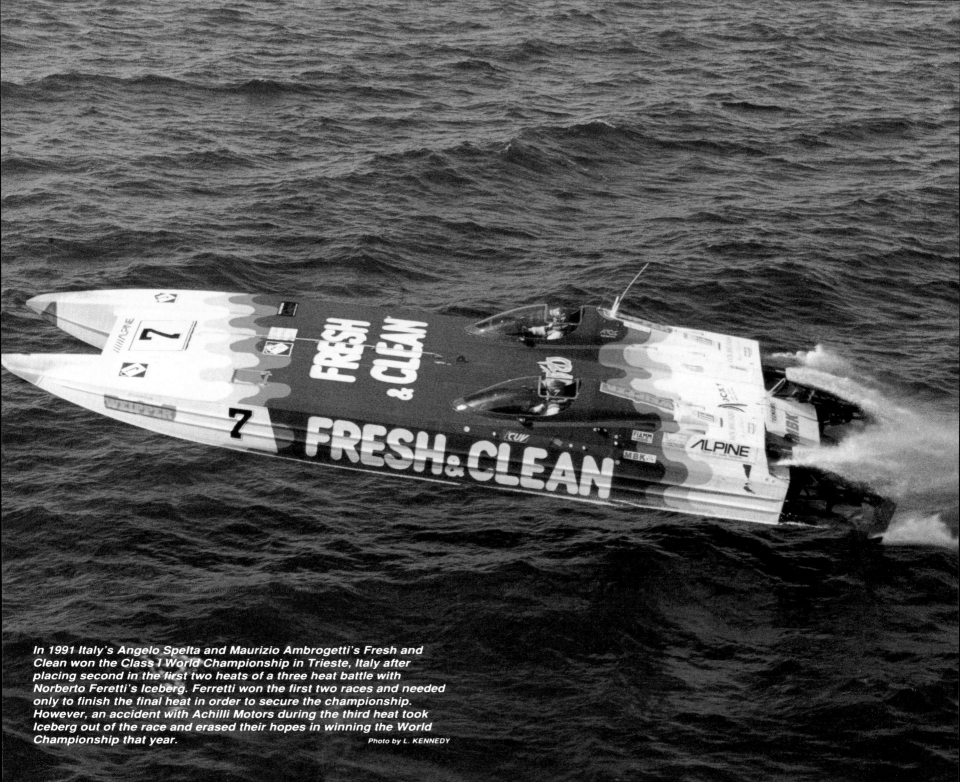

In 1991 Italy's Angelo Spelta and Maurizio Ambrogetti's Fresh and Clean won the Class I World Championship in Trieste, Italy after placing second in the first two heats of a three heat battle with Norberto Feretti's Iceberg. Ferretti won the first two races and needed only to finish the final heat in order to secure the championship. However, an accident with Achilli Motors during the third heat took Iceberg out of the race and erased their hopes in winning the World Championship that year.

Photo by L. KENNEDY

Introducing The Offshore Grand Prix

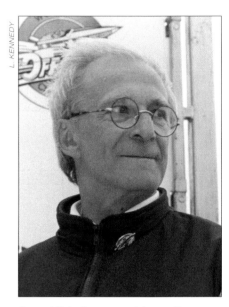

Grand Prix Promoter Mauro Ravenna

Before the end of the 1991 season, both the racers and the organizers of the European Championship could see that Class I had grown beyond its current structure. When looking for an answer to their problems, the answer was provided by Class I promoter Mauro Ravenna in the form of the Offshore Grand Prix.

Remaining under the auspices of the UIM and the UIM rule book, the Grand Prix would be organized and coordinated by Ravenna from his SPES office in Monte Carlo. Ravenna's Grand Prix schedule would spread the nine race season over seven countries, taking advantage of new press possibilities and increasing its value to the sponsors. This enabled international competitors to support their sponsor's marketing needs as easily as the Italians had done in the past.

The Grand Prix concept addressed most of the problems the growing fleet had. In order for Ravenna to guarantee racer turn-out, each team was required to post a $50,000 appearance bond. If they missed a race - for any reason other than those accepted in the rule book - they'd forfeit their bond. At a $50,000 loss, few teams could afford to miss a race, meaning guaranteed competition turn-out, and better sponsorship at races.

With Ravenna running the Grand Prix, SPES would work full time to organize races throughout the world, overseeing their safe operation, professional image and financial commitments. Ravenna's most important job was one that hadn't existed before the Grand Prix: raising sponsorship money and insuring each race appearing on the pre-season calendar actually occurred.

Additionally, SPES would oversee the race site press room, organize press conferences, and develop media and television contracts. The teams would also contribute $30,000 each towards a publicity fund to cover these additional expenses.

With the additional financial requirements demanded of the Class I Grand Prix racer, several things happened. First, those teams who had problems with the financial requirements of Class I before couldn't afford to move up to the Grand Prix. Instead, they retired, merged forces with another team, raced only their national races or returned to Class II. This left only the strongest teams on the Grand Prix.

Secondly, the teams remaining expected increased professional results for the additional expense. With over $80,000 committed to the Grand Prix before they invested a dime on their boats, each team demanded that the problems promoters had in planning an offshore race be a thing of the past. No longer would they stand for cancellation of races, mid-season venue changes, or poorly financed, mis-managed races. The racers had made a commitment to the Grand Prix and expected results in return.

(Right) The Grand Prix's performance bond meant a guaranteed number of the world's best teams at each race site.
Photo by D. LLOYD

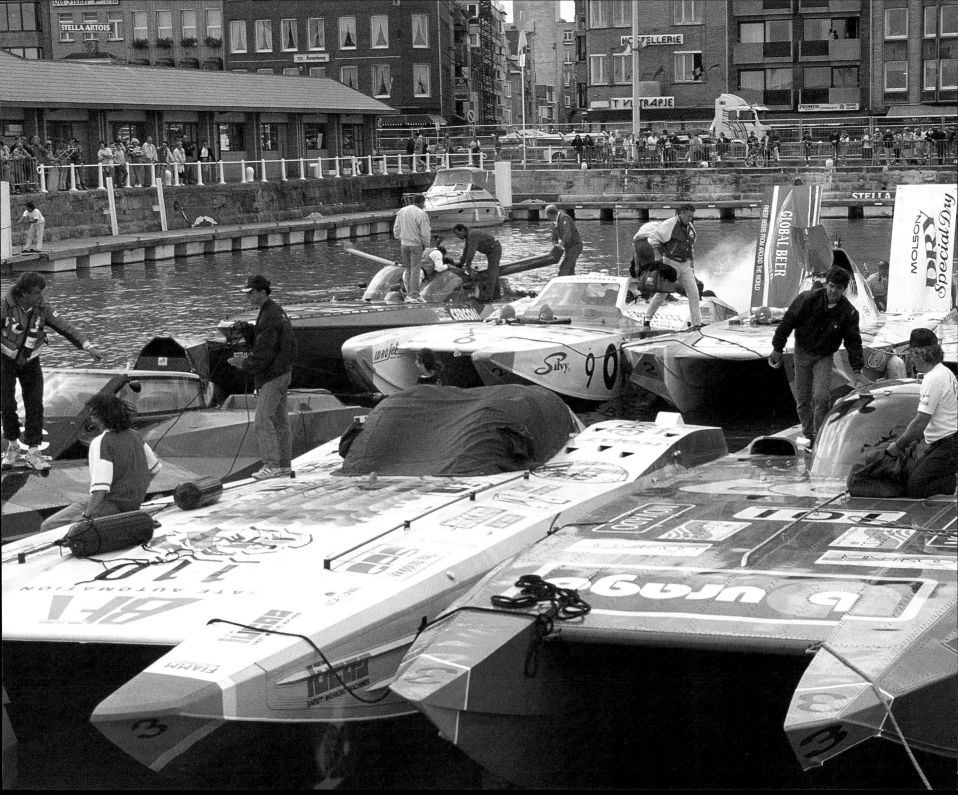

Around the Grand Prix

Each racer must have competed for at least two years (a minimum of 7 events) in their own country before they're awarded the Super License necessary to race on the Grand Prix. Additionally, racers must take a physical examination, provide proof of insurance and pass a dunk test (see Chapter 5) before they compete at Grand Prix level.

At the beginning of the season each team registers the crew and equipment they'll use to earn points towards the World Championship title. Once registered, teams are not allowed to switch crew or boats without loosing their accumulated points. The only allowance made to this rule occurs when a racer or boat has to be replaced because of an earlier accident.

The trickiest pre-season work often involves getting boats to the first race. Transportation of the race equipment isn't easy. In fact, since most boats and trucks average 50-65 feet in length and 10 feet in width, transportation can be quite complicated. For example, Kjell Rokke's *Brooks Shoes*, a 45 foot Skater, was shipped to Europe in the nose of a 747. Once aboard, only six inches remained between the sides of the boat and the plane, proving that even one of the world's largest planes is challenged to transport a Class I boat!

From Europe, the circuit travels from race to race onboard a large freighter. SPES hires a transport company to guard and move the equipment on and off the freighter. Once the freighter arrives at the race site, the teams' truck drivers claim their equipment and head for their pre-assigned spots in the dry pits.

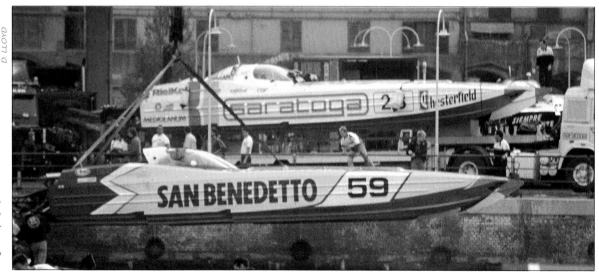

D LLOYD

The pits are a buzz with boats constantly being lifted into the water for testing. Afterwards, boats usually return to their trailers.

The pits are divided into four areas; the sponsor village where teams set up their hospitality areas, the dry pits, wet pits and fueling area. Most of the work on the boats takes place in the dry pits while boats are still on their trailers. Once in the water the boats dock in the wet pits where, like the dry pits, viewing is open to spectators. The fueling area is corded off to keep crowds away from tankers holding the thousands of gallons of fuel to be pumped into the fleet before race day. The fueling area is off-limits to all but registered boat crews.

As crew chief for The Ugland Team, Gianfranco is in charge of their pit crew. Because the boats usually arrive in the pits on Thursday, the pit crew usually has only two days to prepare for the race on Sunday. The crew chief, therefore, has to coordinate a variety of activities in a limited amount of time.

The crew spends Thursdays setting up the hospitality and work areas, cleaning the boat, and checking in with the hotels and race control. The public relations staff shows up on Thursday as well, early enough to set up displays of sponsor materials, make media contacts and represent the team at press conferences. Most of the race teams arrive in town on Friday.

Gianfranco and his crew spend Friday preparing and examining the boat for any damage or minor repair that have occurred during transportation to the race site.

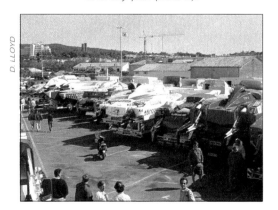

The pits are divided into wet pits (above) and dry pits (below).

Friday is also the day teams report for inspection. The UIM Inspection Commissioner Sergio Abrami and his inspection crew is on hand at every race to make sure each team provides proof of insurance and passes a point-by-point inspection list. Some of the things the inspectors look for are required safety equipment, functioning seat belt releases and correct engine displacement ratios. After the boat has been approved testing of the boat in the actual race waters can be done. The team tests propellers, different "set ups" for the boat and tests all other equipment.

Friday evening the Grand Prix's festivities begin as the boats take to the streets for a parade through the center of town. Teams gladly participate in the boat parades, often inviting local children to join them. Some sites include marching bands, floats, and beauty queens in their parades, while others showcase only the boats themselves. Either way, the Friday boat parade is a fun way to let the public know The Grand Prix is in town.

Saturday morning Andreas and Jann can be found at the Pole Position driver's briefing. The Pole Position Speed Trials run on Saturday afternoon, consisting of a 1/2 kilo run between two marker buoys set up along the shoreline near the pits. Each boat is assigned a turn and clocked as they pass through the marker area. The time they take to pass through the buoys is then used to find their

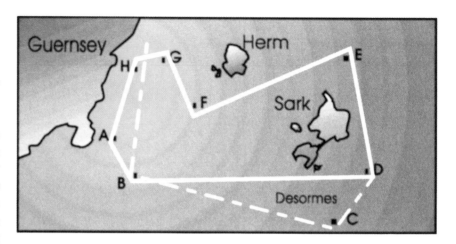

average speed. The fastest boats earn points which are cumulated towards a Pole Position Championship trophy given at the end of the season.

The boat parade and the Pole Positions keep the town excited for the three days of the event and give everyone an opportunity to see the boats up close so they can pick out their favorites. The Pole Positions also give everyone an idea who Sunday's leaders will be. In good conditions boats can log speeds over 130 m.p.h. during the Pole Positions, speeds which cannot be maintained on average throughout a 150 mile long offshore race.

After the Pole Positions teams fuel up their boats and set out to sea for open water testing, go back to their trailers for more work or stay ashore to wait until the start of Sunday's Grand Prix.

The Race Course

Courses on the Grand Prix change from race to race. Some courses are only 120 miles long, others like the Viareggio-Bastia race, almost 160. Naturally, the number of laps coincide with the length of the course. Some courses have only three turns and resemble a triangle in shape, while others have as many as six or eight turns as the course hugs along the shoreline. Courses are announced prior to the race in the driver's circular which is mailed direct to the teams weeks before the event. Specifics to the course are covered at the driver's briefing.

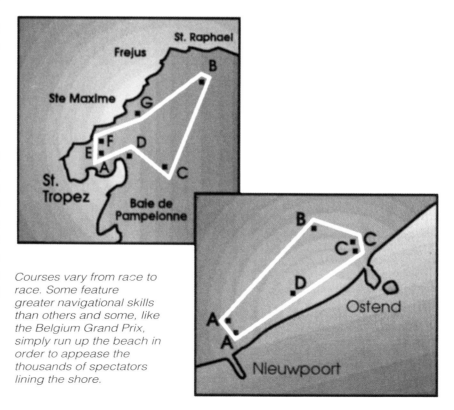

Courses vary from race to race. Some feature greater navigational skills than others and some, like the Belgium Grand Prix, simply run up the beach in order to appease the thousands of spectators lining the shore.

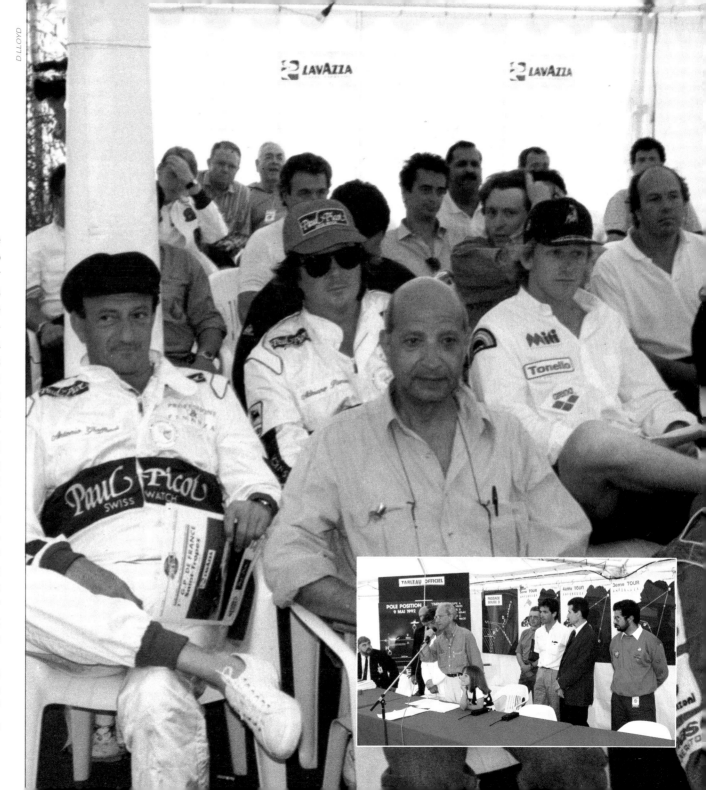

Drivers Briefings

Early Saturday evening the teams attend the first of two drivers briefings for Sunday's Grand Prix. At this meeting, teams are given all the information necessary for competing at that particular race. A large chart of the course is displayed at the front of the room and the local race chairman goes over the course, giving out navigational coordinates, descriptions of turn boats and marker buoys, and the location of spectator fleets. Every detail is carefully covered in both English and Italian. There is no margin for error in navigation. Each boat is scored as they pass the various check points along the course. If a team misses a check point or turns it incorrectly they will not be scored at that point or any points after it. It's as if they were never there.

A final drivers briefing is scheduled the morning of the race to allow announcement of any last minute alterations to the course, and weather conditions.

The Start

The moments before the start of the race are filled with anticipation, excitement and a tension that runs through the fleet like electricity. The boats are ready to race, and now's the time each racer uses to prepare his or herself mentally for the challenge at hand.

Andreas and Jann handle their mental preparation differently. Andreas remains calm and outgoing. He is able to use the time spent in the milling area to garner his focus for the race. Jann, however, prefers to be left alone as much as possible. He is quiet, pulling into himself, centering his energies. He'll usually look over the boat first thing in the morning and then stay away from the crowds until it's time to jump into the cockpit.

Twenty minutes or so before the start, the boats leave the wet pits, heading for the milling area where they'll circle in a counter-clockwise direction while off plane (bow down, no wake), waiting for the Pace Boat to begin the race.

At the milling area, the Pace Boat passes back and forth between two start buoys, indicating where the start line is and holding the boats back behind it. The chief referee, wearing orange gloves and vest over his life jacket, uses hand signals to control the boats prior to the start.

Two minutes before the start a single white flare is fired from the Pace Boat, signifying that the boats can begin their run up towards the start line. Being ready for the white flare is especially important for Andreas and Jann. Because their diesel engines need time to warm up in order to run their best, Jann must get the boat on plane from the far end of the milling area and take a long run towards the start so they'll be at top speed when they hit the start line.

After firing the white flare the Pace Boat displays a yellow flag and heads for the start chute. At this time all the boats go on plane (bow up and accelerating), observing a 30 meter distance behind the Pace Boat.

Once the Pace Boat crosses the start line, the referee raises a green flag, signifying the start of the race. The Pace Boat quickly veers off to the side of the course, clearing the way for the race teams. As the first boat crosses the start line the race is underway. If there are any problems with the start, the Pace Boat would raise a red flag, instructing the teams to return for a restart or go back to the pits for new race instructions.

The start line is a favorite for spectators all along the Grand Prix circuit. The sight of twenty or thirty Class I race boats shooting across the start line, rooster tails and white water flying everywhere, is truly amazing. Boats are lost in the spray of their competitors. The sounds of the engines pouring on full throttle is deafening. And above the boats the sky is filled with helicopters carrying medics, race officials and camera crews.

Everyone watches the start carefully. As the teams wrestle for their place at the front of the pack, some may push too hard and break an engine before the first turn. The start is the only time in the race when spectators can see all the boats together. Once the race is underway, the boats will space out, making it easier to follow the action.

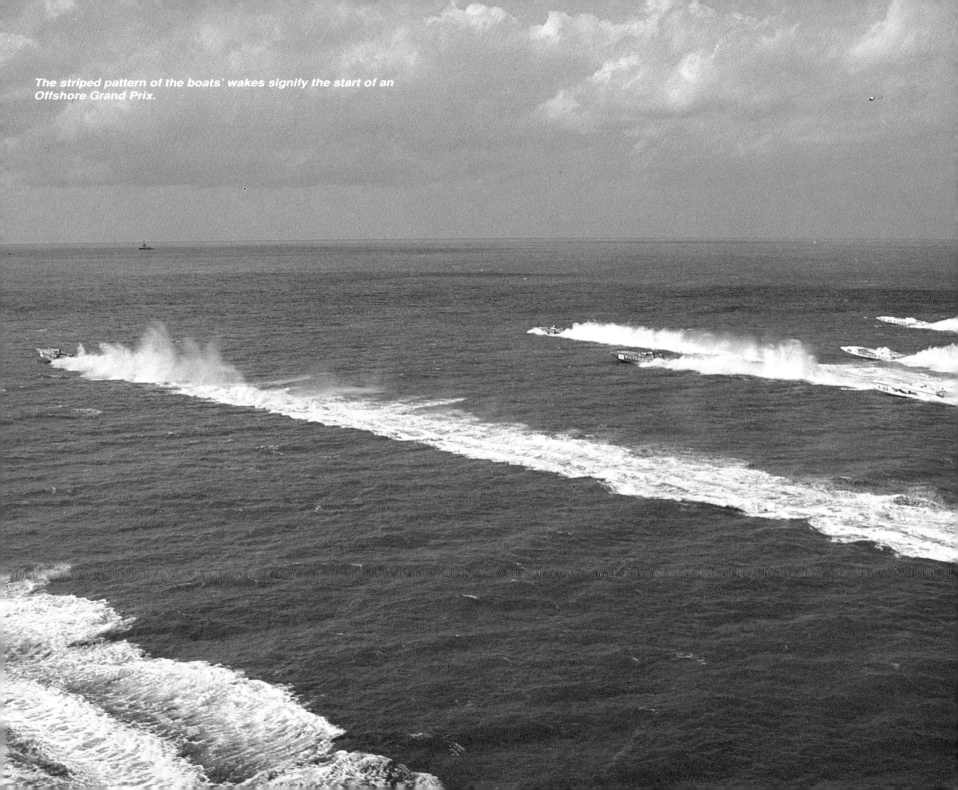

The striped pattern of the boats' wakes signify the start of an Offshore Grand Prix.

The Start From Inside the Cockpit

The start and Turn One are often the most dangerous points of the race. What must it feel like in the cock pit? Jann Hillestad shares his experience by telling the story of the start at the 1993 Ostend, Belgium race.

"The start is very critical for every team. We're all tense, concentrating on what is to come. Sitting just in front of me in the cockpit, Andreas is checking the GPS, charts and stop watches. He'll keep an eye on the old fashioned stop watches to make sure the GPS is working correctly. I start setting the trims for the start. The second set of turbines must be off, the tunnel compressor down, the propeller drives up, the lift aileron in front closed and the trim tabs down a little. If I miss any of these steps, we won't make the start with the rest of the boats.

Slowly we turn in a counter clockwise direction with all the other boats, watching for the white flare. It seems quiet at this time, the only sound being the purr of our engines and an occasional comment over the radio.

Suddenly, a white flare goes up. All the engines roar to life, making is impossible to hear Andreas unless he yells into his microphone. I lower the throttle, bringing the boat slightly up on plane. Andreas avoids the spray of the other boats as he maneuvers us into our best start position.

I keep my focus on the Pace Boat, the throttles and the turbine pressure gauges. Within a few scant seconds the propellers start socking air, and the RPM rises rapidly. With my right hand I control the throttles, with my left I pull slightly back on the turbine throttles, and I use my left foot to trim the tunnel compressor to neutral position. At the same time that I am speeding up, I must stay behind the Pace Boat.

At last the green flag goes up, and we're traveling at about 50 m.p.h.. Now I go full throttle while pulling back the turbine throttles and watching the pressure gauges. We accelerate from 50 to 60 and on to 75 m.p.h. within seconds.

Andreas is watching the other competitors as they pull up alongside us. I push up the turbine throttles to full power. After 2-3 seconds, the engines let out a terrifying surge of torque and we quickly lurch away from the other boats.

"Perfect!" Andreas is yelling out to me over the intercom. "Perfect!" he screams again. Now we are really moving, accelerating to 100, 110, 120, approaching 130 m.p.h. and taking command of the race.

As the speed increases, I'm busy adjusting the trim of the boat. We head for the open sea, shooting across the waves like a bright red arrow.

As we cross in front of the spectators on shore, we know our sponsors and friends are watching us and seeing us out in first place. This makes us even more nervous.

Andreas begins shouting over the intercom again.

"Jann! Come on! Do you have more speed? We're leading! Give me more speed!"

I can't answer him, I'm busy watching the trim at this point. I can't make a mistake or someone will overtake us.

"Jann! Don't you hear me? We're leading! This is fantastic! Give me more speed! Come on!"

"Be quiet!" I yell out to him.

Suddenly the boat hits an unexpected wave, flying out of the water. Andreas holds the steering wheel in place, controlling the boat for the landing. The boat turns on its side while in the air, so Andreas compensates by turning the steering wheel slightly in the same direction. The boat hits the water hard, the impact traveling from my legs all the way through to my wrists. I immediately charge more water into the trim tanks at the front of the boat. Then I lower the trim tabs at the back and get the boat running stable again.

Another large wave follows the first, but we handle this one better. This is the danger of being the leader. The waves shift all around us. We must rely on our ability to read the sea. We can't watch other boats tackle them first.

"I think we're too far out," I yell to Andreas. "Turn left!"

"I can't!" Andreas yells back. Sure enough, several boats have positioned themselves to our left, forcing us out and away from the upcoming turn buoy. Several more waves hit us, slowing everyone down, but Bilba Cadey and Victory 4 sneak past us.

"Jann! I need more speed, we must be in front before the turn buoy!"

"I'm at full throttle. The speed is coming up now. Try to go closer to the inside boat so they'll have to turn out at the turn. We"re still too far out!"

We pull to the inside of the course and can see the turn in front of us. We realize we won't be the first boat into the turn.

"Go wide!" Andreas yells. "Let's take it on the outside!"

I prepare the boat for the turn. Up goes the tunnel compressor, down goes the lift aileron in front. I pull up slightly on the trim tabs and look ahead at the sea and wind conditions on the other side of the turn.

A high speed turn is very risky. Both Andreas and I must coordinate our actions perfectly or we could spin out or barrel roll. As soon as the boat begins to hook, Andreas must release the steering wheel slightly, and at the same time I have to back off the throttles and make sure the turbine pressure doesn't fall too much or we'll loose power.

This time we're lucky. The boat is turning perfectly at over 100 m.p.h. Andreas is switching the GPS to the next navigational point and verifying our position on the chart. I have to set the trims again, open the aileron, put the trim tabs up and charge the trim tanks in front with more water. Soon we're back up to 125 m.p.h. and I set the trim tabs down again so the boat can accelerate in the flatter water conditions.

Andreas begins shouting at me again. "Jann, come on! More speed! More speed!"

I'm trying my best to do ten things at once. "Andreas, please be quiet! I'm at full throttle, but I need to concentrate now. Just wait. I have everything under control."

I start to speed up, but ahead of us the waves are increasing, getting bigger and bigger, challenging all the boats.

What's this? Something is happening! Andreas heads the boat towards an open space and suddenly we are pulling out in front of Bilba Cadey and Victory 4!

"Oh my God!" Andreas is yelling happily. "Look! They're slowing down! They can't keep this speed! What a fantastic day...I love this boat. Come on Jann, let's go for it."

I keep the throttles down while Andreas watches the seas even more intently. On shore our sponsors and friends must be going crazy. Here, inside the cockpit, I have many feelings at the same time. I feel like we're kings of the sea. The boat is running perfectly, and I'm comfortable with the conditions. No one can catch us. This is our water, our day...I'm afraid to hope because I realize there are still over 100 miles left to go."

The Finish

Once clearing Turn One most courses run a long sea leg to Turn Two. Here's where the heavier boats can overtake the lighter ones, as sea conditions toss and turn boats headed out for the next turn. This leg is usually the roughest one. Only the most daring teams go out for first here where they'll have to try and guess an unclaimed sea. The boats will be their furthest away from shore on this leg, making rescue operations more difficult. However, the long sea leg is a strategic point in the race. The first boat in position after Turn Two, if they can keep their boat together, stands a good chance of gaining a greater lead on the inside water and winning the race.

Races usually turn back towards shore for Turn Three, making a triangular course on the outside legs. From Turn Three there may be two to more turns or checkpoints, depending upon the shape of the shore line, or if the course takes the race boats past several busy beachfronts. Races run a minimum of four laps and a maximum of eight laps. The quantity of laps is determined upon the length of the charted course.

Once the first three boats cross the finish line, the race is officially over. The top ten boats earn points for their finish place, with the breakdown as follows:

1st Place	30 points	6th Place	5 points
2nd Place	18 points	7th Place	4 points
3rd Place	12 points	8th Place	3 points
4th Place	9 points	9th Place	2 points
5th Place	6 points	10th Place	1 point

Cruising back into the pits, the first, second and third place teams are escorted to the winner's circle through a welcoming throng of spectator boats. Waiting at the wet pits is a crowd of press, team members and family, all wanting to be the first to interview and congratulate the teams.

After a mandatory one hour delay for official scoring and interviews, the winning teams hop onto an open bed truck for a brief parade through the pits and on to the winner's podium. Soon the champagne is popped and sprayed into the crowd, and the laurel wreaths and trophies awarded at the first of two prize givings. The first prize giving is scheduled an hour after the race for the waiting press and public.

A second ceremony takes place several hours later. This ceremony can be a casual affair for the public or a private dinner for race teams, race volunteers and guests. At the second prize giving another set of trophies is awarded to the race winners as well as the first three teams in Saturday's Pole Positions.

Once the second awards ceremony is over, the event is complete. The tents come down, the race teams leave town and the trucks begin hauling the boats to the freighter where they'll be loaded, dreams and all, to return to their shops for preparation for the next race.

While in between races, the boats will undergo a thorough examination of hull, machinery and equipment. Engines will be opened up, changed, overhauled or renewed depending on their condition. The hull will be examined for any weaknesses and if needed, will be repaired as well.

FINNSCREW

UNOBROKER

GRUPPO UNOHOLDING

8

VILLA D'ESTE

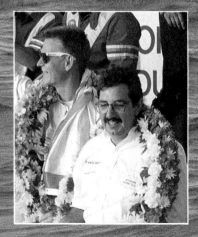

Walter Rigazzi and J.P. Mattila took FinnScrew to the top spot in 1992, winning the first ever Offshore Grand Prix World Championship.

Photos by D.LLOYD

Chapter 3
The Organizers and the Competitors

The race organizers have proven themselves to be as important to the sport as the competitors. Indeed, no event takes place without them. Dedicated professionals, most of the organizers are unpaid volunteers who are only involved for the enjoyment they get from offshore racing.

At the top of the list is UIM President Ralph Fröhling.

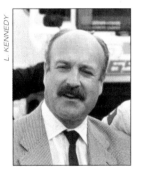

Ralph Fröhling
UIM President.

Covering offshore as well as other UIM racing, Mr. Fröhling coordinates the guidelines of the UIM with the organizers and promoters. Every activity to affect the rules and long term well being of the sport is handled through the UIM; rules, technical specifications, inspection judgements and promotions. Mr. Fröhling serves as the principle representative of the UIM, the man racers can speak to directly.

The UIM Offshore Commissioner and Chairman of the World Offshore Championship is Richard Ridout. Richard is a key player in keeping offshore activities operating within the UIM's regulations. From registrations and driver briefings, to inspections, protests and the general running of the race, Richard is on hand to interpret and enforce the UIM rules.

Inspections are handled by Sergio Abrami, the UIM Technical Commissioner. Sergio trains a bilingual staff in all the technical and safety aspects of offshore boats. Because manufacturers utilize offshore racing as a testing ground for new products, the inspection crews have to work throughout the year to keep

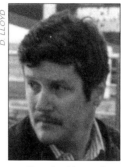

Sergio Abrami
Technical Commissioner.

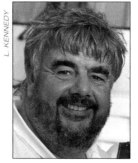

Richard Ridout
Offshore Commissioner.

abreast of the newest technology utilized in offshore racing.

Richard Ridout's right-hand man is David Corsen, another Guernsey native who has dedicated hundreds of hours to offshore. David is a friendly face who is kept busy organizing much of the logistics at the race site. Serving as Officer of the Day at the Guernsey, Ostend and Malta races, David is responsible for supervising official registration, admissions and scoring as well as running the race from the water.

Much of the timekeeping of an offshore race is handled by the local race organizers, but in many instances they rely on scoring expert Colin Le Conte. Colin is a direct assistant to the Officer of the Day, and provides computerised race results within moments of the race, with Lap Position Charts for the top ten finishers, speeds in knots, m.p.h. and k.p.h., the time in seconds, the position each team finished in and the points they earned in the race. Colin also provides immediate updates on the cumulative points earned from all the races and Pole Positions. Come the end of an event, the man most people look for is Colin, the first person to know the official results.

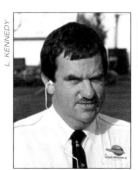

David Corsen
Coordinator.

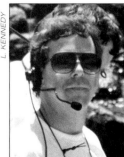

Colin Le Conte
Timekeeping.

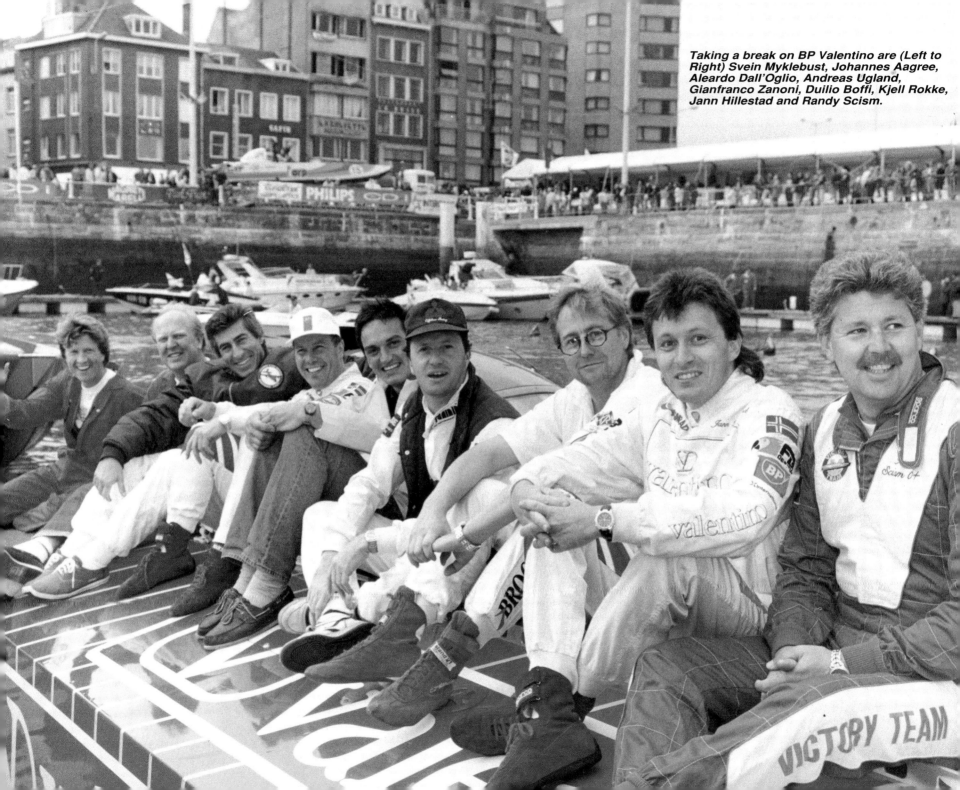

Taking a break on BP Valentino are (Left to Right) Svein Myklebust, Johannes Aagree, Aleardo Dall'Oglio, Andreas Ugland, Gianfranco Zanoni, Duilio Boffi, Kjell Rokke, Jann Hillestad and Randy Scism.

The Grand Prix Competitors

A ndreas and Jann join many other racers who've recognized that one of the best things about racing in Class I offshore is the quality of the people they compete against. Not only is their competition tough and aggressive on the course, but the majority of them are well established international businessmen and women whose intelligence and savvy in their respective fields are what makes it possible for them to compete.

From garment manufacturers, luxury car distributors, yacht builders and appliance company owners to artists and athletes from other sports, the professional background of the offshore competitor is as varied as the colors of their boats. The question is: Why they do it? Why compete in such a dangerous sport when more relaxing ventures are available? The answer for racers at this level seems to be the challenge. Like the man who takes his portable phone to the golf course,

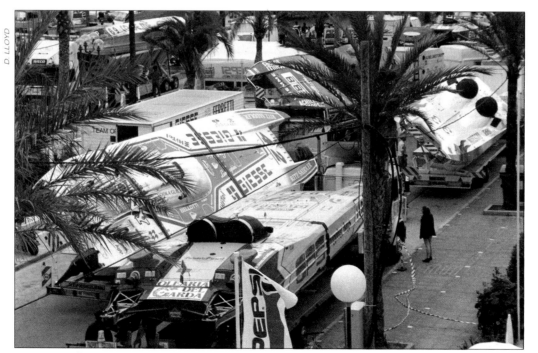

these men and women have a need to keep their brains active, their bodies moving. They find a thrill in the speed of racing, but mainly they flock to offshore for the combination of intense mental and physical challenge, knowing that winning on the race course will never be as easy as the success they find in the boardroom.

Several competitors are professionally paid throttlemen. Included in this elite field are Steve Curtis, Jim Dyke, Randy Scism, Felix Serralles III and Ed Colyer, to name a few.

Several other racers are co-owners of their boat, pooling their funds to purchase a boat, and then funding their racing season through sponsorship.

The 1993 season saw the return of the majority of the teams competing in the 1992 Grand Prix inaugural season as well as new entries from Dubai, Italy and the United States. Overall, 33 different teams competed in the first two years of the Grand Prix. The following pages will introduce you to each of them.

The Grand Prix pits in Marbella are awash of color, power and excitement.

Norberto Ferretti & Luca Ferrari
Giesse - 1992/93

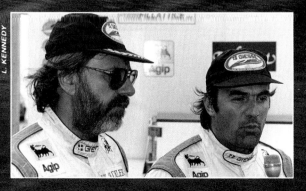

A leader in Class I racing since he first joined the circuit in 1991, Norberto Ferretti came close to being World Champion in both 1991 and 1993. In 1991 Ferretti's *Iceberg* won the first two of the final three heats in the series, suffering an accident in the third. And in 1993 Ferretti's *Giesse* ended the season as the only team close enough in points to upset the domination of the 1993 *Victory Team*. Competing alongside him in the cockpit throughout his challenge was throttleman Luca Ferrari.

GIESSE PHOTO BY D. LLOYD

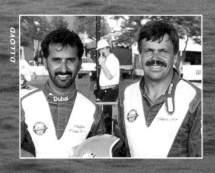

D.LLOYD

Khalfan Hareb & Ed Colyer
1993 - *Victory 4*

It would be hard to recall a team who has had as dramatic an effect on offshore racing as Dubai's *Victory Team*.

Registering three boats on the circuit, the *Victory Team* competes amongst itself as well as with the rest of the field. At the end of the 1993 Grand Prix season any questions as to who was the best among the *Victory Team* was answered when Dubai driver Khalfan Hareb and American throttleman Ed Colyer won four out of eight Grand Prix races, claiming the 1993 World Championship.

VICTORY #4 PHOTO COURTESY OF THE VICTORY TEAM

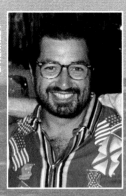

Walter Rigazzi
1992 - *Finnscrew* with J.P. Matilla
1993 - *Kaos Missoni* with Enrico De Marco

VILLA D'ESTE

33

coroner

Walter Rigazzi has never been a man to be underestimated, a point
he made clear in 1992. Racing with Finland's J.P. Matilla, Rigazzi won the
1992 Marbella race, and then garnered enough points to win the first
Grand Prix World Championship title in history.

Returning to the Grand Prix in 1993 with a new sponsor and new
co-driver, Enrico De Marco, Rigazzi raced well, but failed to garnish the
trophies he had the year before. Rigazzi's spirit, however, remains
determined. One World Championship title is not enough for this Italian
competitor.

KAOS MISSONI PHOTO BY D. LLOYD

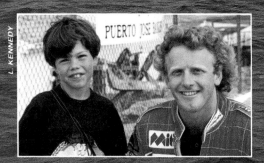

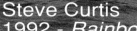

Steve Curtis has long been a favorite with children along the circuit. Here Steve poses with Andrea Ugland III.

Steve Curtis
1992 - *Rainbow Bears* with Leonardo Polli
1993 - *Bilba Cadey* with Lamberto Leoni

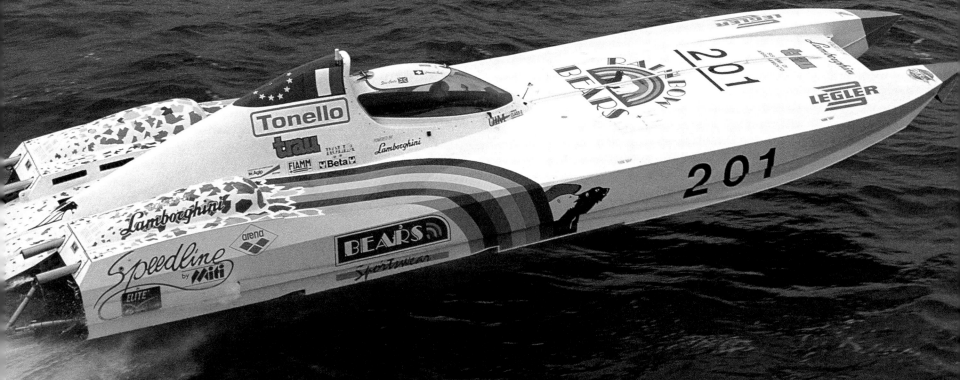

Steve Curtis is a professional throttleman, and one of offshore's most prolific racers. A two-time World Champion himself, there's a saying about Curtis... he's either going to win the race or break the boat trying. This young Brit is known for riding on the edge.

In 1992 Steve Curtis was instrumental in helping Leonardo Polli win the Pole Position Championships. In 1993 Steve was holding down the throttles when Lamberto Leoni took his second win on the Grand Prix, helping secure third place on the World Championships.

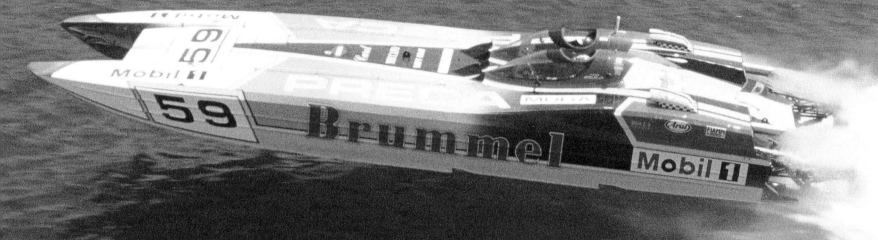

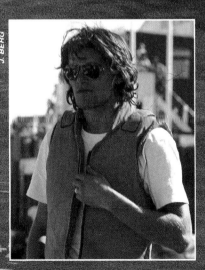

Damiano Spelta & Maurizio Rossi
1992 - *San Benedetto*
1993 - *Preca Moda-Brummel*

The son of 1991 World Champion Angelo Spelta, Damiano is one of the youngest and most intense racers on the circuit. Known for being a hard driven competitor, Damiano believes the only honorable finish is first place. His "take no prisoners" attitude pairs well with his co-driver Maurizio Rozzi, and the two can always be expected to go full throttle for first place.

A World Championship title has, as yet, alluded Damiano. Still, with his spirit and determination, few would be surprised to see this dynamic Italian claim this, his most coveted prize, in the near future.

PRECA MODA-BRUMMEL PHOTO BY D. LLOYD

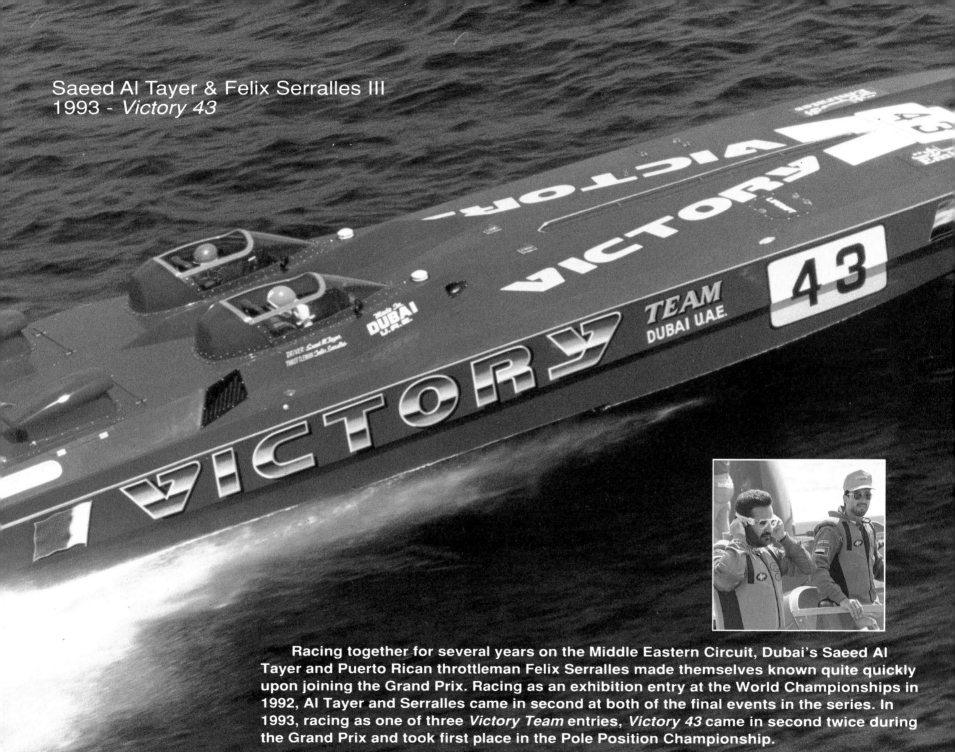

Saeed Al Tayer & Felix Serralles III
1993 - *Victory 43*

43

VICTORY
VICTORY
VICTORY

TEAM
DUBAI U.A.E.

Racing together for several years on the Middle Eastern Circuit, Dubai's Saeed Al Tayer and Puerto Rican throttleman Felix Serralles made themselves known quite quickly upon joining the Grand Prix. Racing as an exhibition entry at the World Championships in 1992, Al Tayer and Serralles came in second at both of the final events in the series. In 1993, racing as one of three *Victory Team* entries, *Victory 43* came in second twice during the Grand Prix and took first place in the Pole Position Championship.

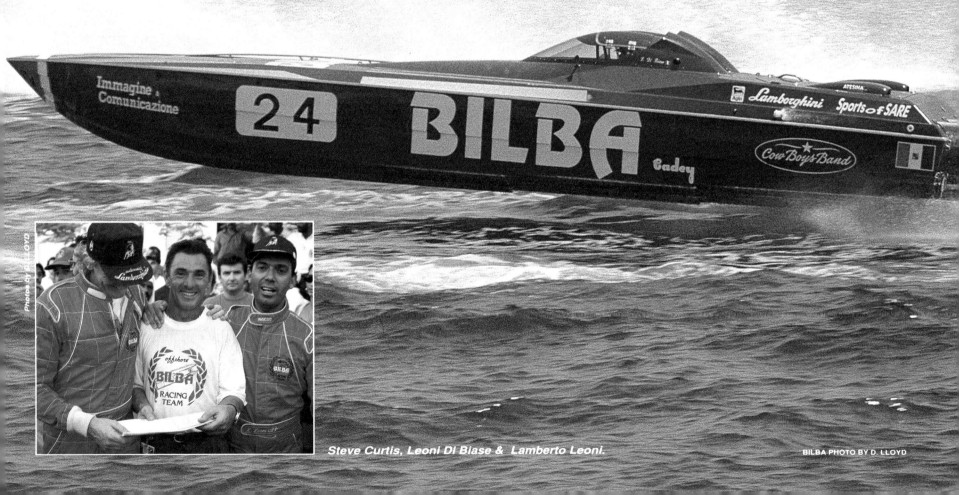

Lamberto Leoni
1993 - *Bilba Cadey*
with Leoni Di Biase & Steve Curtis

New to the Grand Prix in 1993, car racer Lamberto Leoni took to the water as if he'd been racing offshore for years. Starting the season with Leoni Di Biase in the throttleman's position, Leoni won the first Grand Prix race in Marbella. After suffering an accident in St. Tropez, Leoni had to replace his injured co-driver Di Biase, choosing professional throttleman Steve Curtis. Leoni went on to win the Dubai Duty-Free Grand Prix, becoming the only man to beat the *Victory Team* in 1993 and doing it twice for good measure.

Steve Curtis, Leoni Di Biase & Lamberto Leoni.

BILBA PHOTO BY D. LLOYD

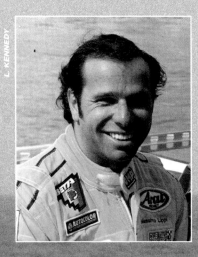

L. KENNEDY

Massimo Lippi
1992 - *Chesterfield* with E. Colletta
1993 - *Fortuna* with Fabio Gera

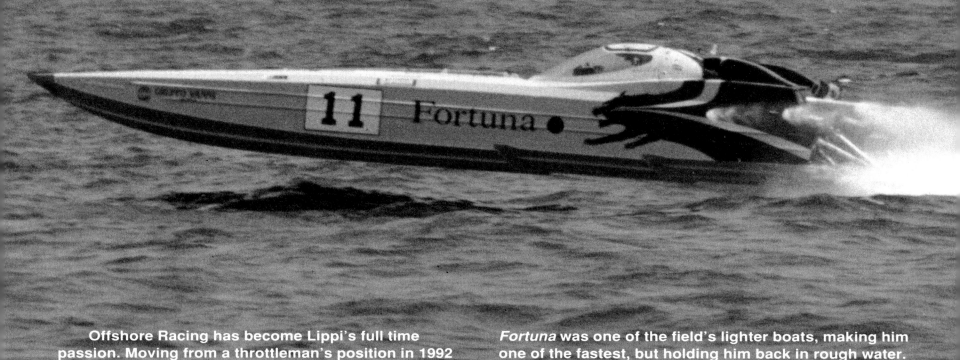

Offshore Racing has become Lippi's full time passion. Moving from a throttleman's position in 1992 to boat owner in 1993, Lippi worked hard in securing a sponsor and in winning races. Quick on the start,

Fortuna was one of the field's lighter boats, making him one of the fastest, but holding him back in rough water.
     Not to be out done, Lippi started plans for 1994 early in 1993, making him one racer worth watching.

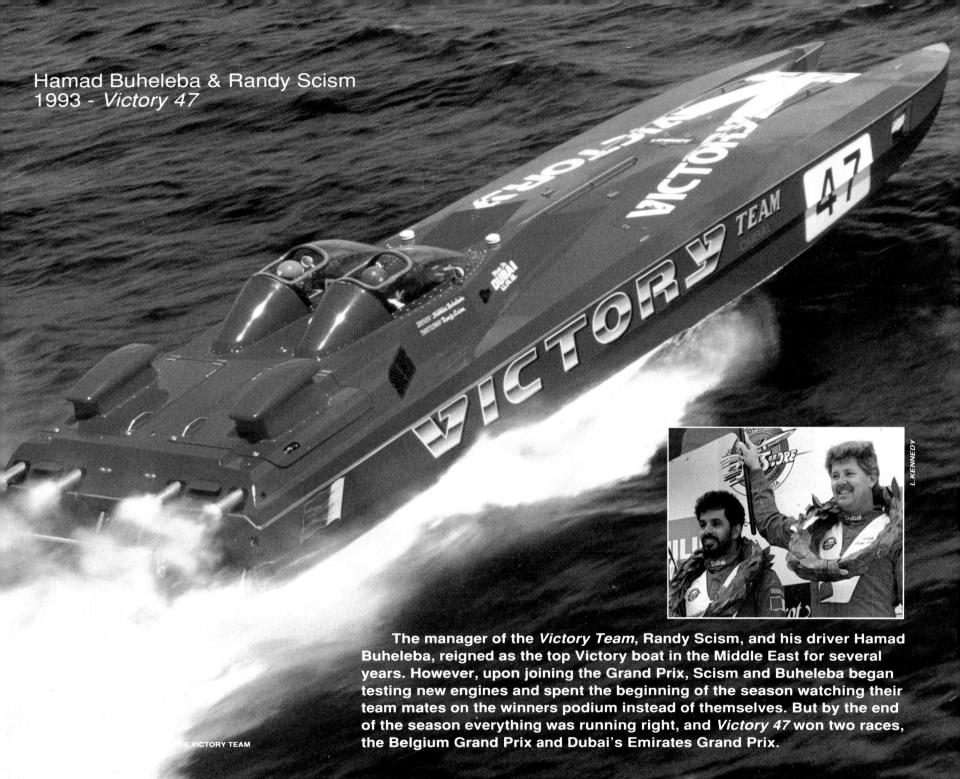

Hamad Buheleba & Randy Scism
1993 - *Victory 47*

L. KENNEDY

THE VICTORY TEAM

The manager of the *Victory Team*, Randy Scism, and his driver Hamad Buheleba, reigned as the top Victory boat in the Middle East for several years. However, upon joining the Grand Prix, Scism and Buheleba began testing new engines and spent the beginning of the season watching their team mates on the winners podium instead of themselves. But by the end of the season everything was running right, and *Victory 47* won two races, the Belgium Grand Prix and Dubai's Emirates Grand Prix.

PHOTOS COURTESY OF ACHILLI MOTORS RACING TEAM

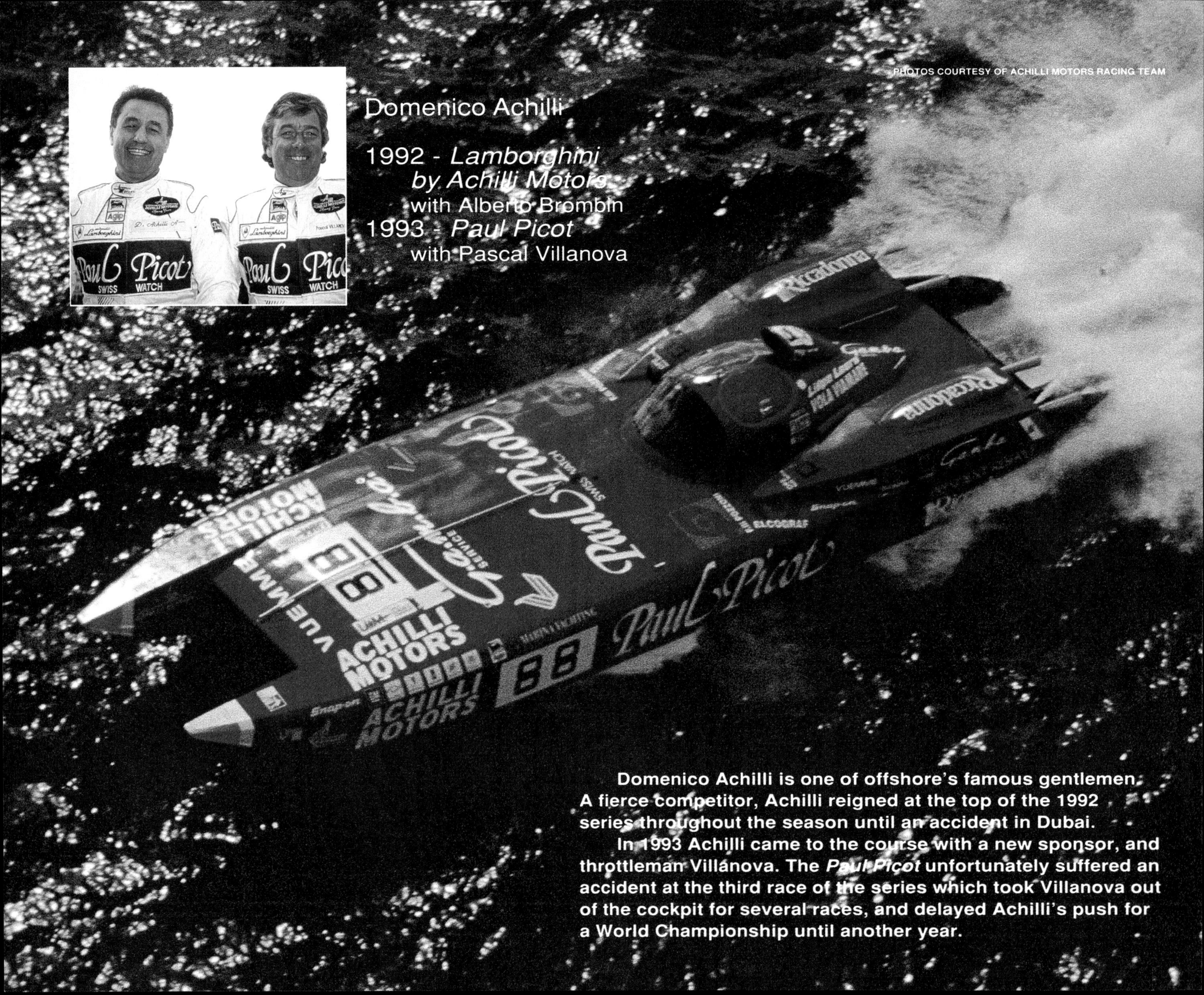

Domenico Achilli

1992 - *Lamborghini by Achilli Motors*
with Alberto Brombin
1993 - *Paul Picot*
with Pascal Villanova

Domenico Achilli is one of offshore's famous gentlemen. A fierce competitor, Achilli reigned at the top of the 1992 series throughout the season until an accident in Dubai.

In 1993 Achilli came to the course with a new sponsor, and throttleman Villanova. The *Paul Picot* unfortunately suffered an accident at the third race of the series which took Villanova out of the cockpit for several races, and delayed Achilli's push for a World Championship until another year.

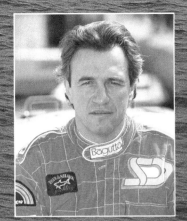

Edoardo Polli
1992 - *SDA* with Vincenzo Polli
1993 - *Rainbow Bears* with Leonardo Polli

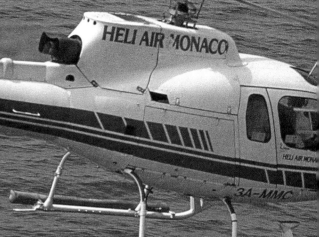

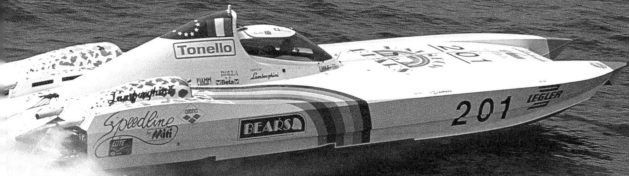

Edoardo Polli's *Rainbow Team* has filled the top winning positions in offshore more than any other organized team. Racing since the early 80's, Edoardo developed his racing talents through the most difficult time in the sport, finally serving as International Offshore Team Association's drivers' representative to the UIM.

Edoardo prides himself in being an innovator, the first to try something new. Early in 1989 Edoardo decided to run a four engine boat, striving for a win until finally achieving his goal at the 1992 Dubai Duty Free Grand Prix. He later wrecked the boat at the very next race, suffering a nasty head bashing in the process. Not giving in, Edoardo introduced a new four engine boat at the 1993 Guernsey Grand Prix, but it caught fire and sank one race later. Unlucky? Not likely. One look at Edoardo Polli's win record dispels that!

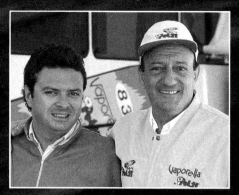

Patrizio Cozzi and Antonio Gioffredi

Antonio Gioffredi
1992 - *Paul Picot* with M. Nicolini
1993 - *Vaporella* with Patrizio Cozzi

Gioffredi was probably the first European to run a composite hull and the first to race a trimaran on the Grand Prix. The winner of the 1992 Pescara Grand Prix, Gioffredi suffered one of the most horrific accidents caught on film when *Vaporella's* engine broke loose in an accident, tearing through the side of the boat, and crushing the legs of both drivers. Gioffredi was back at the races in Dubai, two months later. Turning sixty during the 1993 Grand Prix season, he admitted he just could not retire without first winning a World Championship title.

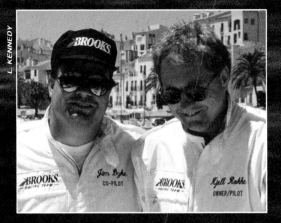

Kjell Rokke & Jim Dyke
1993 - *Brooks Shoes*

Joining the Grand Prix in 1993 as the reigning U.S. Class I National and OPT World Champions, Rokke and Dyke were quick to assimilate to the level of competition offered in Europe. Taking a third place finish at the Guernsey Grand Prix and a fourth in the St. Tropez Grand Prix, the duo was intensely serious in their search for a win. Rokke and Dyke remained one of the season's most competitive throughout 1993 even after suffering a chilling roll-over accident in Malta.

BROOKS SHOES PHOTO COURTESY OF KR RACING TEAM

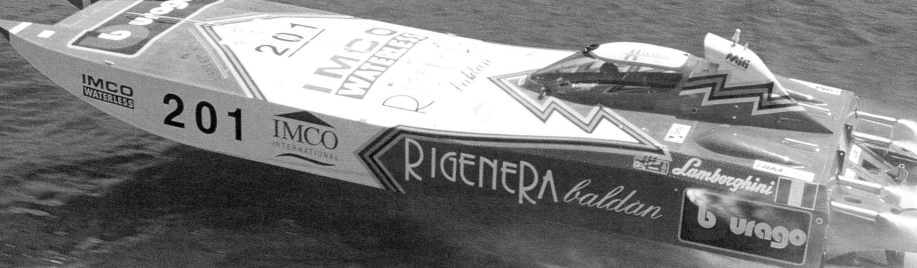

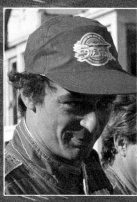

Vincenzo Polli
1992 - *SDA* with Edoardo Polli
1993 - *Rigenera Baldan*
    with John Balzarini

Vincenzo Polli started racing under the guidance of his uncle Edoardo, and raced two seasons with Steve Curtis. With the introduction of the Grand Prix in 1992, Vincenzo returned to driving for Edoardo before switching to the throttleman position and beginning a new racing partnership with Balzarini in 1993.

A successful racer in his own right, 1993 was uneventful for the *Rigenera Baldan* team, a fact which set well with both men. Vincenzo was just learning the throttleman's position, so the duo preferred that he save his aggression until he'd earned more race time in that occupation.

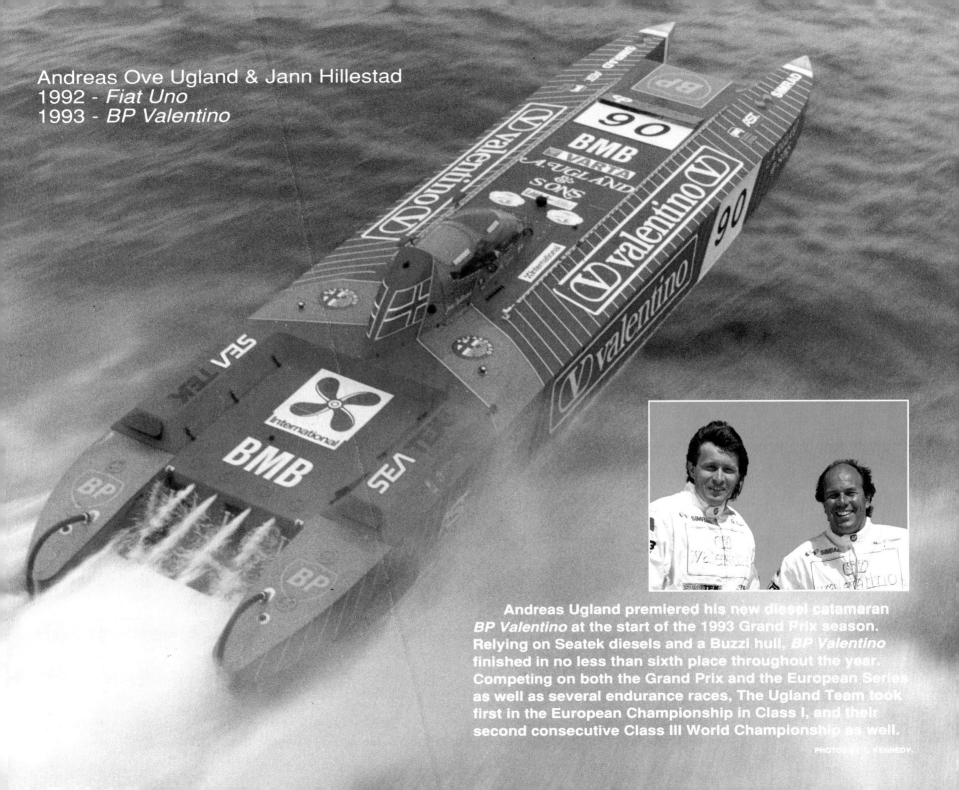

Andreas Ove Ugland & Jann Hillestad
1992 - *Fiat Uno*
1993 - *BP Valentino*

Andreas Ugland premiered his new diesel catamaran *BP Valentino* at the start of the 1993 Grand Prix season. Relying on Seatek diesels and a Buzzi hull, *BP Valentino* finished in no less than sixth place throughout the year. Competing on both the Grand Prix and the European Series as well as several endurance races, The Ugland Team took first in the European Championship in Class I, and their second consecutive Class III World Championship as well.

PHOTOS BY L. KENNEDY

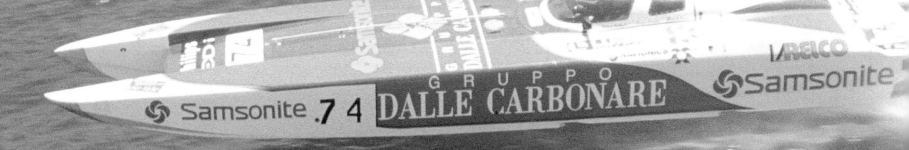

Jacopo Carrain
Gruppo Dalle Carbonare
1992 with Paolo Patergnani
1993 with Aleardo Dall'Oglio and Dirk DePauw

Carrain consolidated his efforts in the 1993 season by joining forces with Aleardo Dall'Oglio, and adding Belgium's Dirk DePauw as navigator. The boat ran well both seasons, but Carrain's crowning moment on the Grand Prix was being the official points winner of the Emirates Grand Prix in 1992.

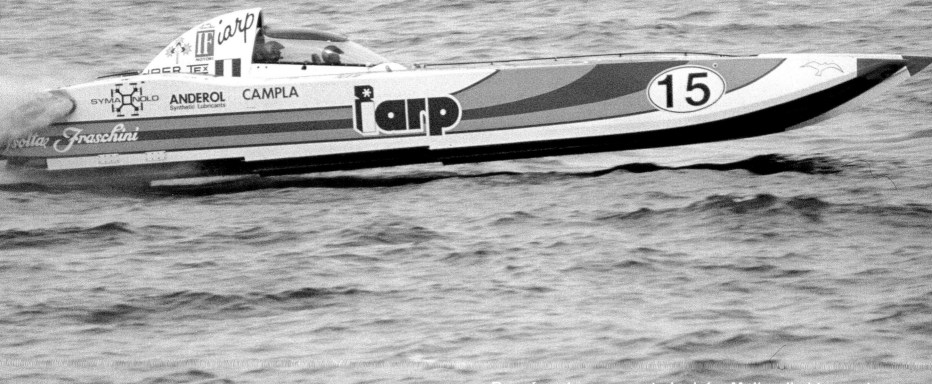

Renato Molinari & Carlo Bodega
1992-93 - *IARP*

IARP PHOTO BY D. LLOYD

Race fans have come to look for Molinari's blue and white *IARP* wherever they expect to find world class racing. A World Champion with one of the longest racing careers behind him, Molinari is a true sportsman who not only races boats, but also builds them. His co-driver Carlo Bodega has raced with him through to the end of the 1993 Grand Prix season.

Renato Luglio - Giancarlo & Monica Rampezzotti
1992 - *Johnny Lambs*
1993 - *Eberhard*

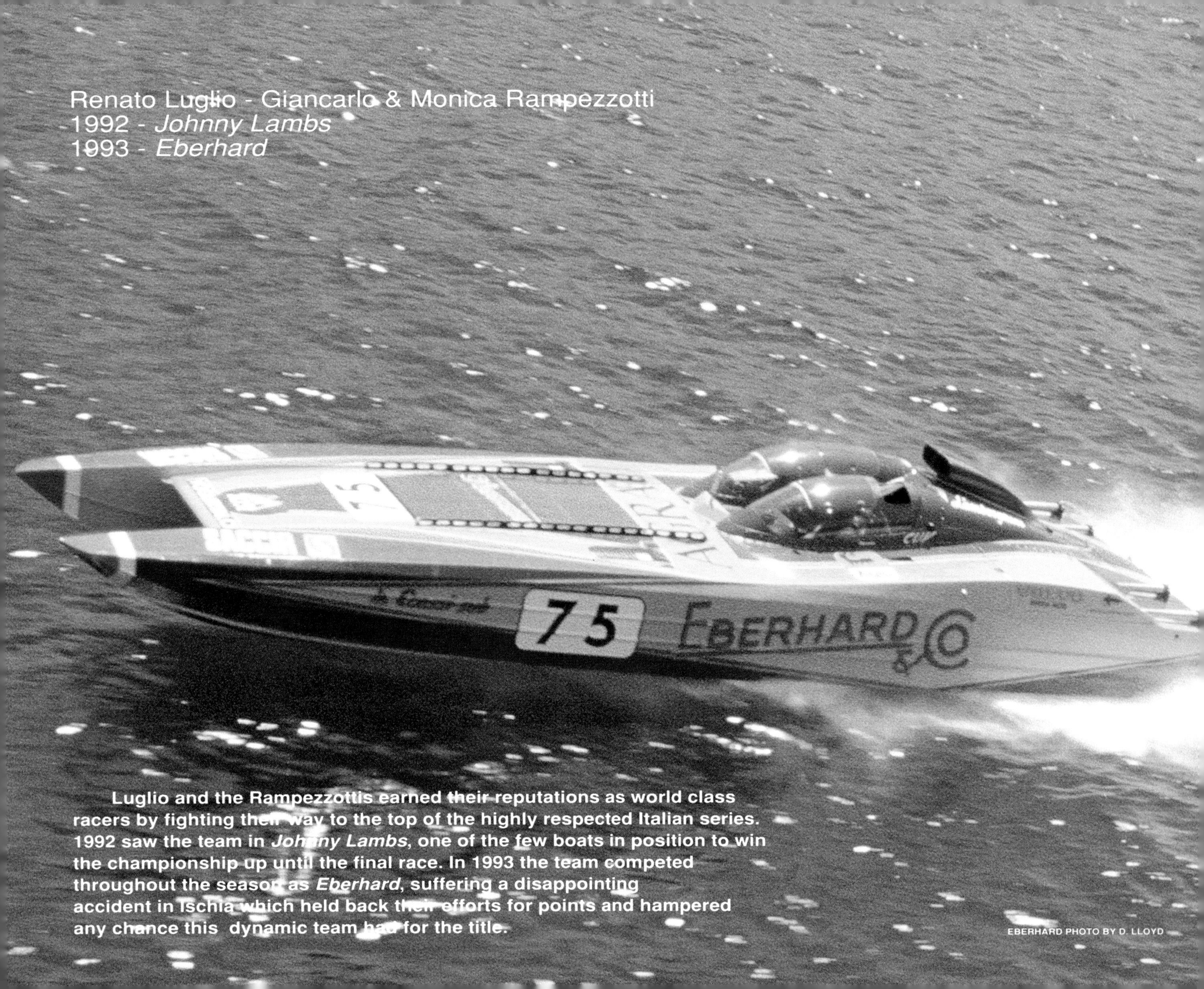

75

EBERHARD & CO

Luglio and the Rampezzottis earned their reputations as world class racers by fighting their way to the top of the highly respected Italian series. 1992 saw the team in *Johnny Lambs*, one of the few boats in position to win the championship up until the final race. In 1993 the team competed throughout the season as *Eberhard*, suffering a disappointing accident in Ischia which held back their efforts for points and hampered any chance this dynamic team had for the title.

Massimo Rugarli
1992 - *Bindi Fantasia* with B. Guarracino
1993 - *Vodka Glaciale* with Adriano Panatta

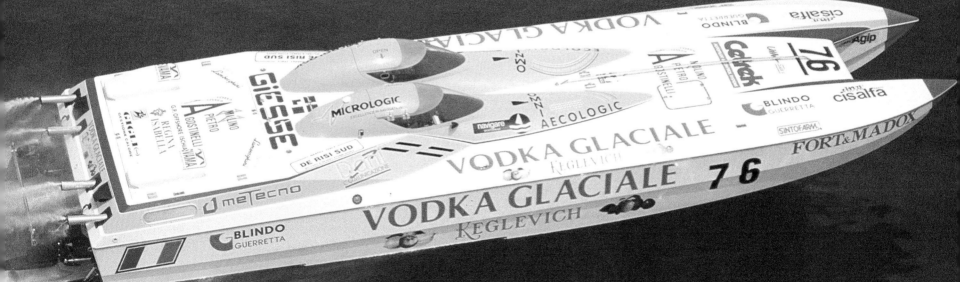

Rugarli enlisted a new sponsor in 1993, and a new throttleman. Whichever of the two made the difference, Rugarli became a points earning team in 1993. His *Vodka Glaciale Ferretti* showed increasing promise as the season went on, seeming to gather ever increasing speed as Rugarli grew more comfortable with the abilities of his throttleman Adriano Panatta. Panatta is well known in the professional tennis world and equally respected in offshore powerboat racing.

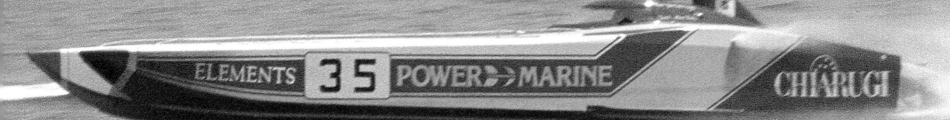

Giancarlo Corbelli & Alberto Diridoni
1993 - *Powerboat Marine #35*

ELEMENTS 35 POWER MARINE CHIARUGI

Corbelli is the owner of *Powerboat Marine*, and therefore the sponsor of two boats. His stronger entry was *Powerboat Marine #35*, the winner of two heats in the '93 Pole Position competition and holder of the fastest kilo run of the season, 127.54 mph. His throttleman, Diridoni, has been racing since 1970 and holds an enviable record in long distance racing as well.

Duilio Boffi
1992 - *Frattelli Rossetti Velmont* with Alessandro Zocchi
1993 - *Pepe Jeans Velmont* with Paolo Patergnani

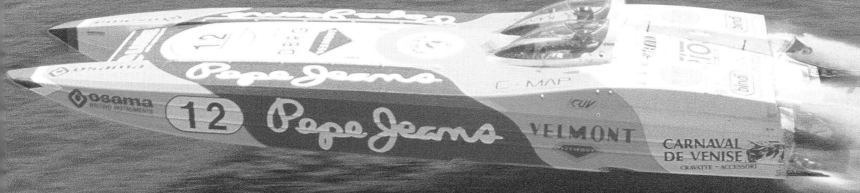

Boffi has always proven to be a strong contender on the course, a man whose obvious enjoyment of the sport never fails. Finishing in seventh place overall in 1992, Boffi was plagued with mechanical problems throughout 1993. Not to worry, though, Boffi and Patergnani still gave it their best at every race, enjoying themselves thoroughly all along the way.

PEPE JEANS VELMONT PHOTO BY D. LLOYD

Sergio Chiarugi & Roberto Biancalana
1993 - *Powerboat Marine #34*

The duo of Chiarugi, an Italian fashion industrialist, and Biancalana, a boat builder, has shown strong potential since first racing together in 1993. Chiarugi has been racing Class I since 1991, and Biancalana, throttleman for the team, has experience racing in both Class I and Class III. This mix, plus a stubborn desire to win, made the *Powerboat Marine #34* entry a positive contender in 1993, their fresh spirit giving them even greater promise for the future.

POWERBOAT MARINE #34 PHOTO BY G.P. HAGEN

Domenico Cirilli
1992 - *Paul & Shark* with M. Riganti
1993 - *Sant'Orsola* with Serafino Barlesi

POLOARTICA 20 S. ORSOLA ASTI SPUMANTE

   Racing in 1992 in *Paul & Shark,* Cirilli was an important member of the Rainbow Team, and one of the season's leading boats. Cirilli branched out on his own in 1993, racing in *Sant'Orsola*. The move has yet to reward him, coming from sixth place overall in 1992 to land in the top ten only one time during 1993. Those knowing Cirilli realize they can expect more from this hard driven racer in the future.

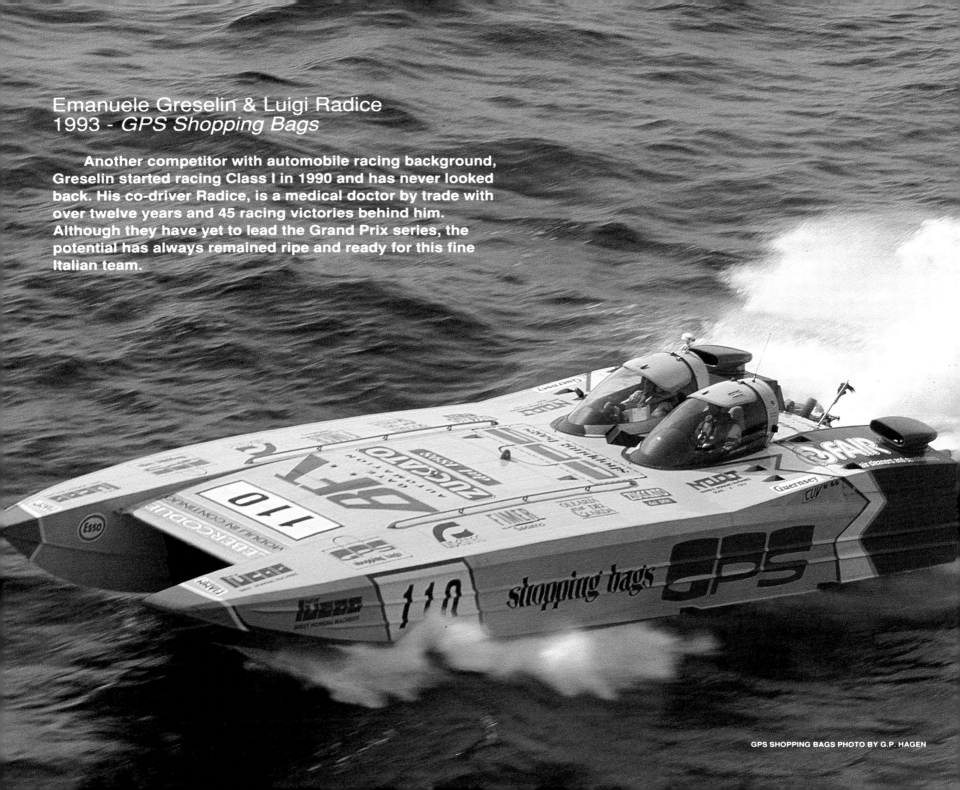

Emanuele Greselin & Luigi Radice
1993 - *GPS Shopping Bags*

Another competitor with automobile racing background, Greselin started racing Class I in 1990 and has never looked back. His co-driver Radice, is a medical doctor by trade with over twelve years and 45 racing victories behind him. Although they have yet to lead the Grand Prix series, the potential has always remained ripe and ready for this fine Italian team.

GPS SHOPPING BAGS PHOTO BY G.P. HAGEN

Didier Puccini & Gian Luigi Coletti
1993 - *Macef*

The only team to list Monaco as home, the *Macef* team of Coletti and Puccini are a colorful duo indeed. An ex-car and motorcycle racer, Coletti seems continually drawn to dangerous sports. His co-driver Puccini, who broke his arm racing in St. Tropez in 1992, doesn't seem to worry about pain either. He jumped into the cockpit a few races later in Guernsey, had a stuffing accident, and was still coming back for more in 1993.

Francesco Pansini & Floriano Omoboni
1993 - *Cogeme Iteco*

Although Pansini and Omoboni never made it to the winner's circle in 1993, no other team garnished the international headlines as the duo did in Guernsey. Running the boat up onto the rocks on Friday, the team still made the start on Sunday, only to suffer a accident which left Pansini in the hospital fighting for his life. Once recovered, both Pansini and Omoboni were back in the boat in Dubai attempting to make the headlines again, only this time with a win.

COGEME PHOTO BY D. LLOYD

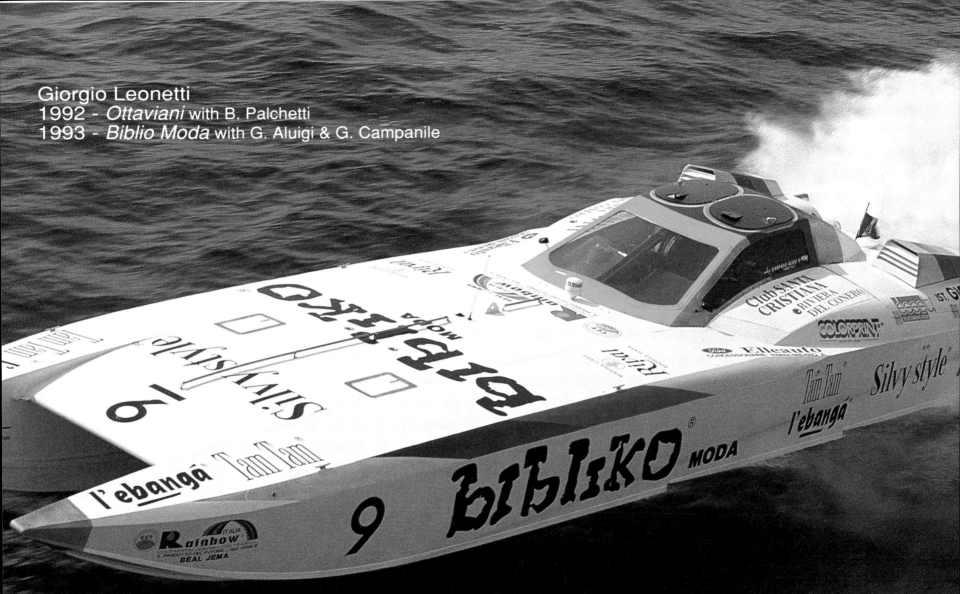

Giorgio Leonetti
1992 - *Ottaviani* with B. Palchetti
1993 - *Biblio Moda* with G. Aluigi & G. Campanile

Giorgio Leonetti is another racer who refuses to give in to defeat. For several years, Leonetti's brightly colored catamaran has registered and raced in Class I but has yet to win. His jump into the Grand Prix seems to have helped, for as his sponsorship value increased there were those willing to put their money behind this competitive racer.

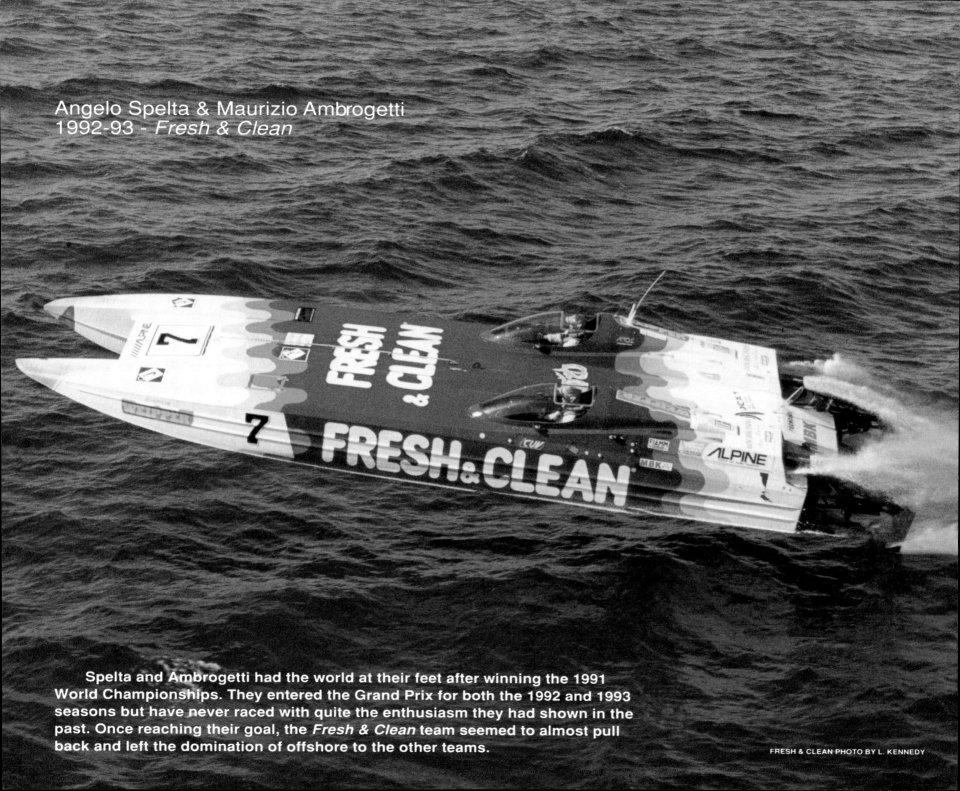

Angelo Spelta & Maurizio Ambrogetti
1992-93 - *Fresh & Clean*

Spelta and Ambrogetti had the world at their feet after winning the 1991 World Championships. They entered the Grand Prix for both the 1992 and 1993 seasons but have never raced with quite the enthusiasm they had shown in the past. Once reaching their goal, the *Fresh & Clean* team seemed to almost pull back and left the domination of offshore to the other teams.

FRESH & CLEAN PHOTO BY L. KENNEDY

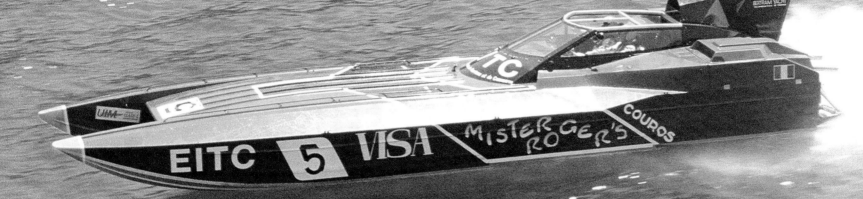

John Pierre Frutiew & Bruno Palchetti
1993 - *Mister Rogers*

Although the boat *Mister Rogers* may have outlived its worth in offshore racing, its team has not. Plagued with troubles at each and every race in 1993, Frutiew and Palchetti continued to appear at each event and attempt to at least make the start. An expensive venture at best, the duo's spirit still shows a team strong in competitive urges.

Massimo Capoferri
1992 - *Passlunch*

The eldest son of Marco Capoferri, Massimo has proven to be a strong racer as well. Earning his chance to race Class I in his own boat by securing both strong finishes and a sponsorship in Italy, Massimo competed on the Grand Prix for the 1992 season where he finished in the top ten four times. He did not return for the 1993 season.

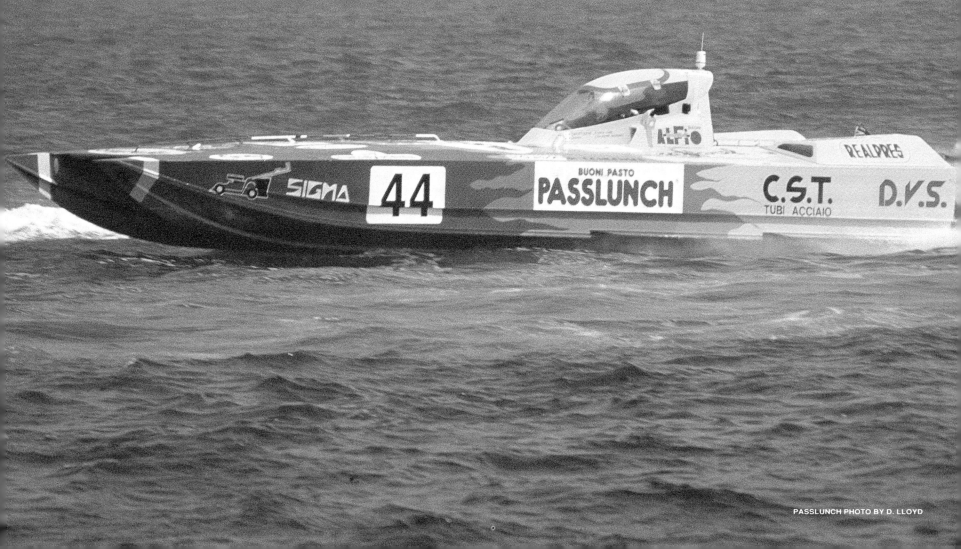

PASSLUNCH PHOTO BY D. LLOYD

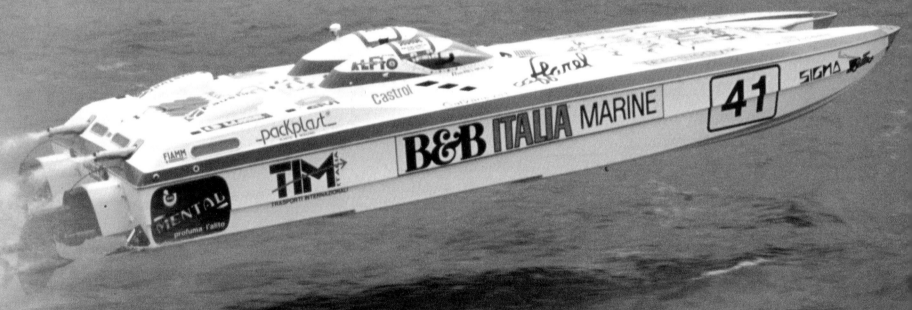

Marco Capoferri & Pierluigi Rivolta
1992 - *B & B Italia*

B & B ITALIA PHOTO BY L. KENNEDY

Capoferri's strong business sense told him that the Grand Prix could have been even better than it was during its first season, and consequently pulled out from the series to run the European Championship. The series continued on successfully without him, though his willingness to speak out has been missed. Capoferri became the European Champion in 1992 and took second on the European series in 1993.

Richard Carr & Peter Dredge
1992 - *Tekne Lamborghini*

Carr ran Class I in 1991 as well as the first season of the Offshore Grand Prix. A strong contender from the start, it was a small shock when Carr decided to bow out from international competition to concentrate on his businesses in England. Still, within his two year career in Class I, Carr became known for his strength on the course as well as his boisterous activities and practical jokes on land.

TEKNE LAMBORGHINI PHOTO BY L. KENNEDY

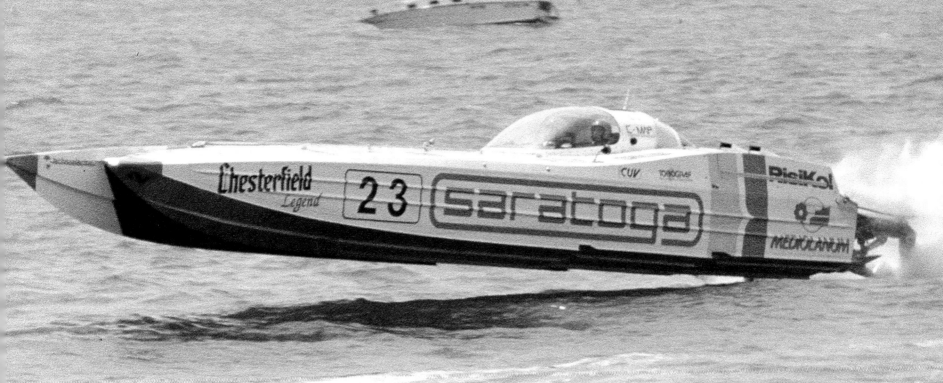

Gianni Arnaboldi
1992 - *Saratoga*

An Italian fashion industrialist, Gianni Arnaboldi's *Saratoga* was a keen competitor in 1992, though Arnaboldi failed to return to the Grand Prix in 1993. Although a recession may have held this racer back in Italy to concentrate on business, many consider his energy and determination to be one of the ingredients that made 1992 a successful year for the Grand Prix.

Chapter 4
Winning the Technology Race

The technology surrounding offshore powerboat racing is as changing and unpredictable as the sea. A case in point: In the 1980's many of the Class I boats resembled standard factory hulls. Fans could walk through the pits and pick out a Cigarette or Apache hull, a standard Cougar or a Skater. Those same fans would find themselves challenged to do the same in the pits of the Grand Prix today. Many teams opt for custom built hulls, and guard their boat's blue prints like a state secret. Others utilize factory hulls, but their race canopies, rigging and custom aerodynamics change the look of the hull almost beyond recognition.

So what should you as a spectator know about offshore technology in order to follow a race? Nothing, really, if all you're interested in is the excitement, speed and final outcome of the event. However, knowing the basics of offshore technology is like having the inside track at a race. Understanding how a boat runs can enable you to predict last minute alterations to a boat's set-up when teams

The difference between the two basic hull designs are shown above and on the facing page. Above, is the Fiat Uno monohull. The bottom of the boat is one hull which comes to a v at the line of center.

need to accommodate for changing sea conditions, wind or air temperature. Recognizing how a boat is supposed to look when running at correct trim can warn when a team has lost an engine, trim tab or drive. Knowing the difference between the sound of a petrol Lamborghini and Seatek diesel can send spectators an advance audio signal of which team is approaching, often before they are visible. Knowing what kind of hull each team is running will tell you which boats can safely run a high speed in rough water and which boats will be hard to catch on flat seas. Technical knowledge can only add to the enjoyment of watching an Offshore Grand Prix.

A brief overview of the basic technology involved in offshore racing follows. Some technology is not covered, but only because explanation of those mechanics is too detailed or does little to enhance spectator viewing. What is covered is the most basic, the most important - standard hull construction and design, canopies, air intakes, drives, navigation and engines.

Hull Designs

Not too many years ago most of the boats in Class I were aluminum or wood, an even mixture between catamarans and monohulls. However, all that changed with the onset of carbon fibres in hull construction. Monohulls have long been favored for their strength and stability in rough water, catamarans for their lighter weight and speed in smooth water. However, when built of aluminum even the catamarans were heavy, at least until builders like Jaguar, Skater and FB Design switched to composite hulls built of Kevlar and carbon fibers. Now the catamaran was not only lighter, but also stronger.

Unlike aluminum boats, which are bolted together along seams, composite boats are formed in layers into a mold, coming out as one solid piece. This single form design makes the hulls stronger with less weak points. They also absorb shock better and can be patched quickly after an accident.

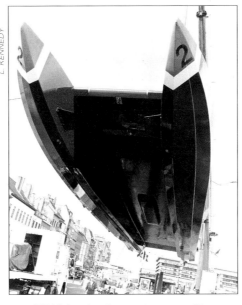

BP Valentino is a catamaran. Two sponsons under the boat are connected by the deck to form a wind tunnel which lifts the boat over waves. Also visible at the front of the under-deck is the hydraulic tunnel flap, which drop down to decrease the depth of the tunnel.

Because they are made as one piece, different technology can be accommodated on composite boats. When Fabio Buzzi designed Ugland's new 1993 catamaran, *BP Valentino,* he knew the boat would be lighter than the team was used to. Therefore, Buzzi designed an air flap under the deck which allowed Jann to decrease the depth of the tunnel while racing, reducing the force and lift of the wind under the boat. This allowed the boat to hold proper racing trim (a term which applies to the angle of the boat as it glides across the water) and decreased the opportunity for the wind to build up under the boat, lift it out of the water and possibly flip it over.

Other details to watch for in hull design is the team's choice in length and beam (width) for their boat. Shorter boats are often lighter and speedier, but less stable in rough seas. Wide boat are stable, but less aerodynamic. Longer boats can reach across most waves, but take more horsepower to achieve top speed.

Canopies

One of the technological advances that makes the most sense and is most fascinating to spectators are canopies. Looking over the fleet, one can witness that no two canopy designs are identical. There are tandem cockpits, split cockpits with driver and throttleman racing side-by-side in separate cockpits, single cockpits with a crew of two racing side-by-side under one canopy, and the larger cockpits, such as that seen on *Giesse*, allowing three to four crew members to race under one canopy.

The purpose of the canopy is to protect the team. In an accident where any part of the boat becomes submerged or hit by water, the force of the water travels up along the deck and *over* the canopy, never actually hitting the drivers. Offshore canopies were originally taken from F-16 fighter aircraft, but boat racing canopies now exist as well.

Regardless of cockpit design, there are actually two types of canopies - the fully enclosed canopy, such as seen on *BP Valentino* and *Fiat Uno*, and the open canopy, seen on all three *Victory Team* boats. Use of one style of canopy over another is a matter of choice. Some teams prefer the quiet of the closed canopy and the knowledge that water can't enter the cockpit until the canopy is opened. Others prefer the open canopy because it is cooler and they like knowing they can exit the cockpit quickly without concern over a possible jammed canopy hatch. At this time of this writing, neither canopy has shown significant merit over the other.

At right, the twin canopies of Fiat Uno, Ugland's 1992 Grand Prix boat, shows enclosed hatches with handles both on the inside and outside of the cockpit.

Photo by G.P. HAGEN

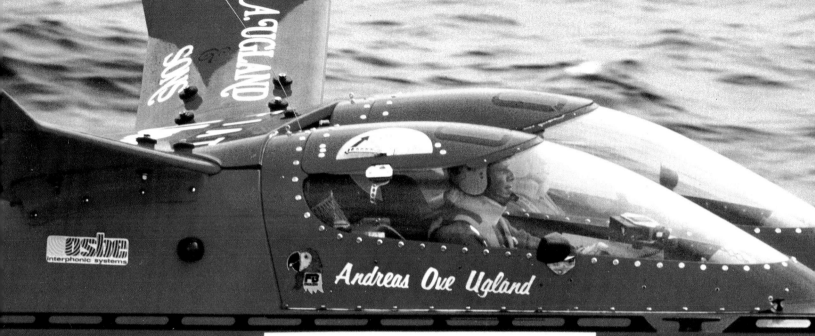

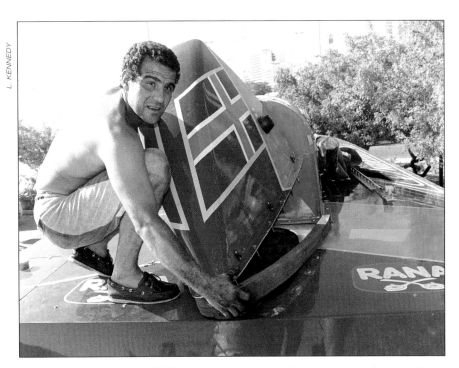

L. KENNEDY

Mauro, a mechanic on BP Valentino, re-attaches the air scoop after creating a new, three inch high gasket to increase air intake.

Air Intakes

Each boat has air intakes toward the back of the deck, often on the engine hatches, which bring cool air into the engines. Air intake designs can be as varied as the boats themselves. Buzzi designed a large air intake directly behind the tandem cockpit of *BP Valentino,* large and high enough to scoop in sufficient air to cool the engines while still following the aerodynamic curve of the cockpit. As the boat races along the waves the curve of the deck forces on-coming wind up and around the cockpit, right into the air intakes and on into the engines. Buzzi's single intake design proved valuable to the team later in the season, as it allowed a quick modification at the warm water races in Dubai. Because the Grand Prix runs in cooler water throughout much of Europe, the hotter air and water conditions in Dubai caused many of the boats to overheat early in the first race. When *BP Valentino* fell victim to this problem, the Ugland crew was quick to find an alternative. Taking off the air intake, Gianfranco's men cut a new three inch rubber gasket to run along the bottom edge of the air intake, lifting it an additional three inches. Ice could then be stored in the bottom of the intake tunnel, cooling the air before it reached the engines.

Many of the other teams utilized new, stylish air intake designs as well. The most notable were those of the 1993 *Victory Team.* After testing new intakes on *Victory 43* in 1992, all three *Victory* boats switched over to them at the start of 1993 season. *Victory's* intakes consisted of two air scoops 'mushrooming' up on top of the engine hatches directly over the engines. This design must take into consideration the team's need to run hard races throughout their own hot, arid Middle Eastern season.

Propellers

I t is exciting to be in the pits just before a race, specifically during those split seconds before boats need to be in the milling area. Especially if crews need those last few seconds to change propellers.

The wind tends to change throughout the day, and a severe change in wind strength or wind direction can result in sea conditions dramatically different from those the team may have tested in only hours before. When that happens the pits explode into a rush of activity as crews rush back and forth from their work trucks, changing props on boats waiting to be craned into the water, and even those already in the sea.

Most teams carry several sizes of propellers, small for rough seas, large for calm water and the new five blade propeller for mixed sea conditions. Each size propeller has its own attribute and plays an important part in determining the rate of speed a boat can maintain while racing.

Because propellers are so important some race sites, such as Dubai, have developed on-site propeller tuning stations in their dry pits so teams can dial in necessary changes to their propellers right before a race. At the propeller station edges are ground to precision and any nicks suffered during testing are evened out.

Propellers have also been instrumental in showcasing the strong level of sportsmanship on The Grand Prix. A good case in point involves the 1993 Ostend, Belgium race when Steve Curtis, throttleman for *Bilba Cadey*, was seen rushing through the pits in a panic. The wind conditions had changed, and *Bilba* was left short in their choice of props. Curtis went to Kjell Rokke,

the owner/driver of *Brooks Shoes*, whose boat was also a 40' Skater. Anyone familiar with Rokke knows there isn't a more determined racer on the circuit. Rokke wants to win, and doesn't hold back anything in his determination to champion the circuit. *Bilba* had already won one race and was high up in the point standings. Rokke's *Brooks Shoes* was rapidly moving up in points as well and stood as good a chance as any to win the Ostend race. If *Bilba* ran the wrong props, *Brooks Shoes* would have an advantage over one of the top contenders. Yet when asked for a set of props, Rokke not only loaned Curtis the props, but also rushed him back and forth through the pits on his scooter so *Bilba* could be ready for the start.

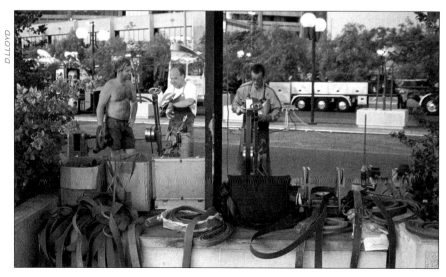

Belts, grinders and race crews work to get the boats race ready in the Dubai dry pits' propeller station.

The Drives, Trim Tabs and Tie Bars

The drive system connects the power generated by the engine to the propellers. The rudder and propeller shafts are considered part of the drive system. There are a variety of drives used in offshore, but the most famous names are Kiekhaeffer, Mercruiser, Trimax, BPM and Arneson.

The drive system is very important to the over all performance of the boat. So important, in fact, that in the weeks prior to the unveiling of *BP Valentino,* Fabio Buzzi was consumed with thoughts on how he could improve the boat's drive system. Fabio kept himself and his mechanics working overtime on the drives for the new catamaran. Once his original drives were installed, Buzzi went home to sleep, confident that he had come to a good solution. Yet that night he dreamt of an even better system, one which would allow the drives to be trimmed not only left and right, but also up and down. He hopped out of bed, re-designed the drives, and had the mechanics ripping out the old drives the moment they reported for work the next morning.

The trim tabs and tie bars are very important in determining how the boat handles, but are also the two areas on the boat which seem to suffer the most breakage. Trim tabs are the small, hydraulically driven "steps" at the bottom back of the hull. (They are easily seen on the top two pictures on the next page). Trim tabs are controlled by the throttleman, and are instrumental in setting the angle at which the boat rides on the water. Wind and water conditions can over-ride the setting of the trim tab, and cause the boat to run off center in unexpected conditions. A particularly hard bounce against the sea can actually break a trim tab, causing the boat to run off balance, forcing it to stop or slow down.

Tie bars are the long metal bars connecting the drives at the back of the boat. The tie bars sole responsibility is to ensure that the drives and rudders are working in synchronization. If a tie bar breaks a boat can veer out of control as the rudders aim off in different directions.

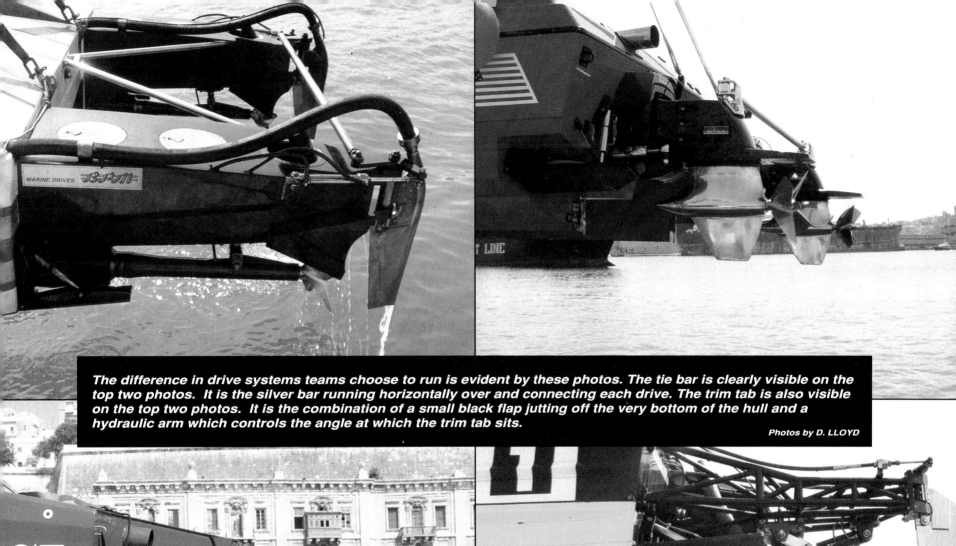

The difference in drive systems teams choose to run is evident by these photos. The tie bar is clearly visible on the top two photos. It is the silver bar running horizontally over and connecting each drive. The trim tab is also visible on the top two photos. It is the combination of a small black flap jutting off the very bottom of the hull and a hydraulic arm which controls the angle at which the trim tab sits.

Photos by D. LLOYD

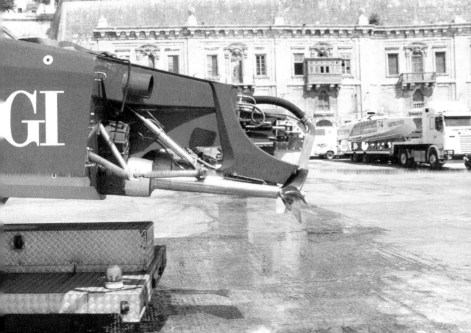

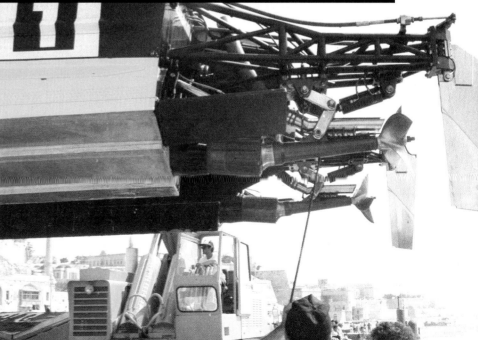

The Question of Power

Taking all technology into consideration nothing is more impressive than the engines of an offshore boat. Their sheer size is a marvel to first time spectators. Averaging over 1,200 lbs each, a single engine is approximately three feet high by three feet wide and about four feet in length. Most boats utilize two engines, some use three, while Edoardo Polli's *Rainbow Bears* uses four.

The number of engines used has never been a major question in racing, Polli has been one of the few to test four engines. The real subject of controversy on engines is the diesel v.s. petroleum question. Engine limitations in Class I are 1,000 cubic inches on petrol engines (16.39 liters) and 2000 cubic inches on diesels (32.78 liters). As late as 1990 the majority of the European boats ran diesel engines, but in 1993 the ratio showed signs of a reversal. Sixteen of the '93 Grand Prix entrants ran petrol engines, ten ran diesel.

The leaders in the petrol engines have been the Lamborghini and U.S. Sterling engines. The Lamborghini are the more famous, known for their tell-tale whine, while Sterling racked up the most wins. Also showing strength in European racing is the Mercury engine, which is popular on the United States racing circuits but has only recently shown serious intent on the Grand Prix.

In the diesels engines, there were eight Isotta Fraschini diesel boats and only two Seatek. However, the Isotta's quick starts didn't hold Seatek's reliability or lower expense.

Costs involved between petrol and diesel engines give the petrol team a price advantage. Although petrol engines tend to be rebuilt more often than diesels, they are less expensive in the long run. The reliability of the diesel, which made it the engine of choice when offshore teams raced far from shore, doesn't play as important a roll on the Grand Prix where courses are shorter and close to shore.

The diesel's past history of being slow on the start was always a question, one which both Seatek and Isotta Fraschini answered in recent years, giving their teams enough start power to lead several of the Grand Prix's first laps. The Isotta Fraschini powered *Powerboat Marine #35* was consistent in its first lap attempts to grab a spot at the front of the pack, and even won two pole positions during the 1993 season, scoring the fastest pole position speed of the year, 127.54 m.p.h.. *BP Valentino* won the St. Tropez pole positions in Malta at 126.22 m.p.h. and broke two world speed records in December, 1993, setting a new Class I record of 145.16 m.p.h. and a new Fondo World Speed Distance record of 103.49 m.p.h..

The 1993 World Championships, however, went to Sterling engines, in both the Grand Prix races and in the Pole Position competition. So, although diesels have shown they're every bit as fast as petrol engines, the 1993 Grand Prix was still won by petroleum powered boats which may cause even more teams to continue switching over to petrol.

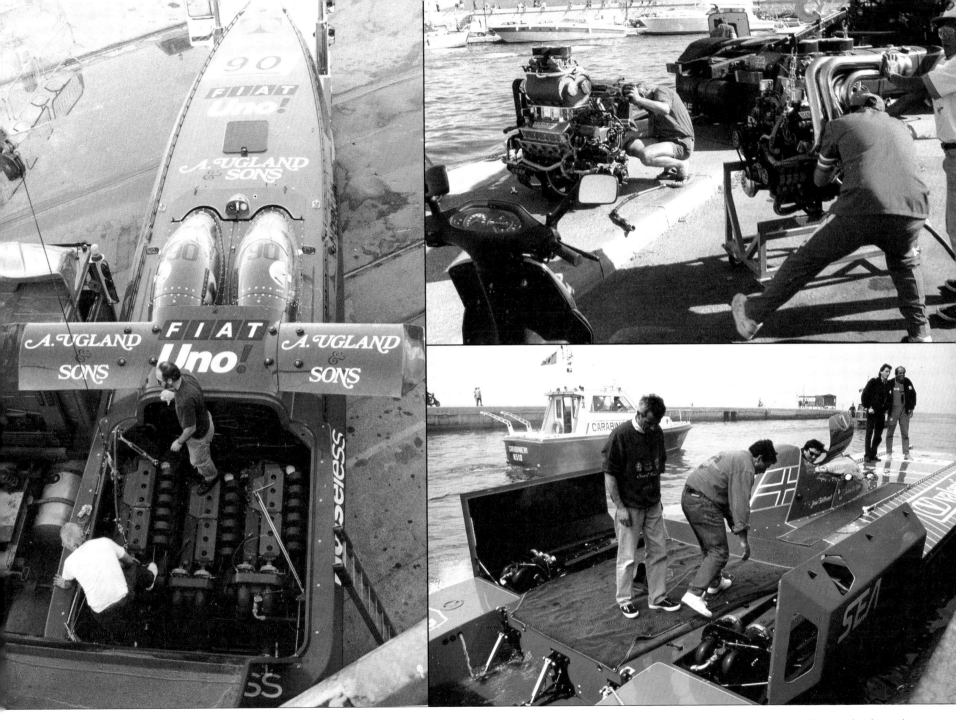

ABOVE: Fiat Uno carried three Seatek engines in one central engine compartment. TOP RIGHT: The Victory Team's Sterling engines were impressive in and out of the boat. BOTTOM RIGHT: BP Valentino's two Seateks rode in separate engine compartments.

Victory Team photo by D. LLOYD, Fiat Uno and BP Valentino photos by L. KENNEDY

Gauges and Navigation Equipment

I f you look inside the cockpit of any race boat you'll be interested to learn which team member controls the various equipment and gauges while racing. The division of controls responsibility may change slightly from team to team, but most teams rigg their boats much the same.

Since the driver does much of the navigation, the compasses and speed gauges will be the driver's responsibility. Much of the mechanical and engine gauges are then covered by the throttleman.

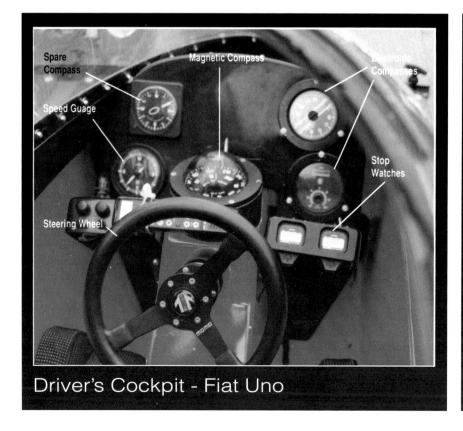

Spare Compass

Magnetic Compass

Electronic Compasses

Speed Guage

Stop Watches

Steering Wheel

Driver's Cockpit - Fiat Uno

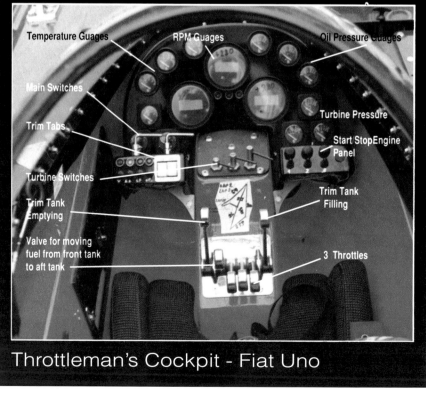

Temperature Guages

RPM Guages

Oil Pressure Guages

Main Switches

Trim Tabs

Turbine Pressure

Start StopEngine Panel

Turbine Switches

Trim Tank Filling

Trim Tank Emptying

Valve for moving fuel from front tank to aft tank

3 Throttles

Throttleman's Cockpit - Fiat Uno

Photos by L. KENNEDY

The Five Dollar Part

For some reason, no race is ever completed without at least one team breaking down due to the loss of the infamous "five dollar part". Although the parts themselves may run more than five dollars, the term has come to represent the variety of small parts from sea strainers, to clamps and hoses that, when broken, can take a team out of the competition.

There are no pit stops in offshore racing. If a team returns to the pits, they are deemed out of the race. So, loss of a "five dollar part" is probably the most discouraging thing to happen to a team, especially since so many parts are small enough that teams could carry extras on the boat and are accessible enough that repairs could be made while the boat is still on the course. Rules mandate, however, that teams can't carry extra parts that could become projectiles during an accident and injure the racer. In reality, there are really too many of these "five dollar parts" to carry anyway.

Yet time after time teams and their crew chiefs can be seen looking over a broken clamp, a torn hose. Often these parts blow out towards the end of the race, usually to a leading boat that is pushing harder than the part can bear. The "five dollar part" illustrates the difference between pushing hard enough to win, and hard enough to break. Consequently, it is not unusual to see a boat with a substantial lead slow down on their last lap. It's not because they want their competitors to catch up... it's because of the "five dollar part" - the one reason even a leading boat doesn't feel safe until they're given the checkered flag.

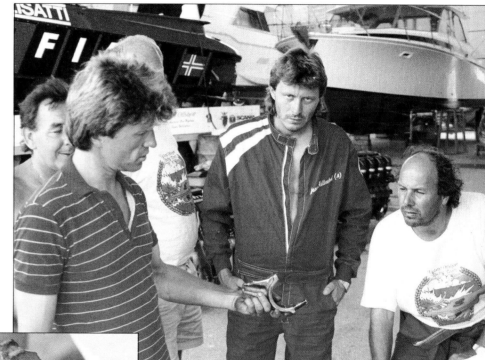

Above and left: The term "five dollar part" applies to any small part that can break and take a team out of a race, even though the part may cost a great deal more than five dollars. In these photos Svein Myklebust displays the "five dollar part" that took Fiat Uno out of the top position at the Venice to Monte Carlo endurance race in 1992. The broken part, a connecting rod, holds the piston to the crank shaft.

Photos by L. KENNEDY

Chapter 5
Surviving the Sea

Racing involves risks, especially boat racing, because no one can ever predict the sea. Speeding towards a turn buoy, each team must be actively calculating the degrees of the turn, the angle at which their boat can handle the turn, how fast they can enter and exit the turn, the location of other boats in the turn, the location of spectator and official boats, the direction of the wind and the swells of the sea. Complicated? Definitely, so it goes without saying that anyone who can't handle these kinds of pressures should not be racing.

The number of safety measures taken on the race course and the number of safety devices built into offshore boats has increased dramatically since the beginning of the decade. Many of these safety measures and devices were incorporated after the UIM and the US American Powerboat Association studied films and wrecks of previous accidents.

Seven Kinds of Accidents

It has been determined that there are seven different kinds of accidents occurring in boat racing. The first type of accident is called the *barrel-roll* which, as it sounds, involves the boat rolling side over side horizontally before stopping. If a team is lucky the boat will roll over deck side up, making it easier for them to exit the boat.

The second kind of boat racing accident is called the *blow over* or *kite*. This type of accident is pretty much unique to catamarans. In a *blow over*, a significant amount of wind gets under the tunnel of the boat (the space under the deck between the two sponsons) and lifts the boat straight up on its transom, flipping it over on its deck. In a *kite*, the boat will lift up, but fall back down into the water without blowing over. If the boat lands

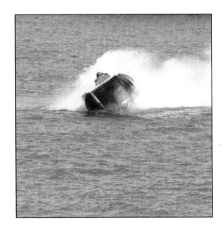 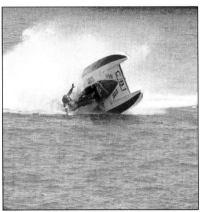 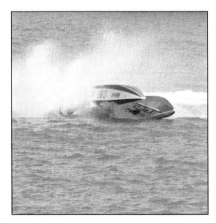 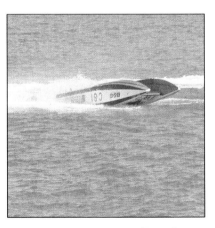

The above photos illustrate a barrel roll. Note that the sponsons do not hook or catch the preceding wave. Please also note that, because these Class II competitors did not utilize a canopy, both racers were ejected from the boat.

Photos by D. LLOYD

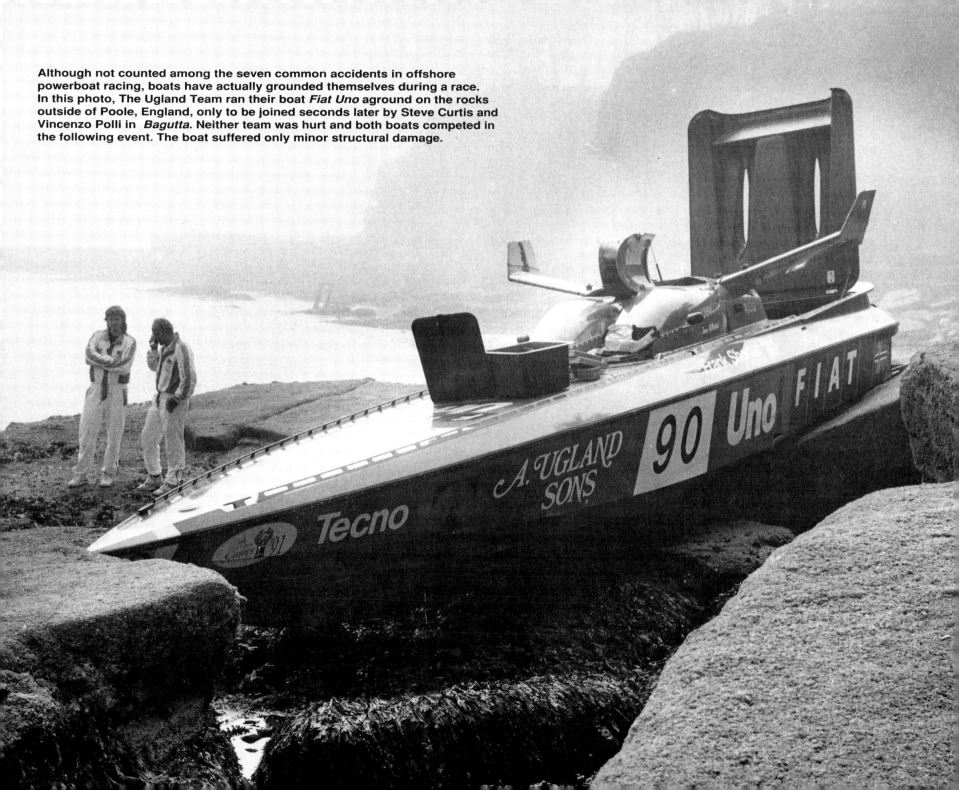

Although not counted among the seven common accidents in offshore powerboat racing, boats have actually grounded themselves during a race. In this photo, The Ugland Team ran their boat *Fiat Uno* aground on the rocks outside of Poole, England, only to be joined seconds later by Steve Curtis and Vincenzo Polli in *Bagutta*. Neither team was hurt and both boats competed in the following event. The boat suffered only minor structural damage.

straight down on its transom, there is the danger that the force of impact will push the engines up through the hull of the boat.

The third type of boat racing accident is the *hook*. The *hook* involves the boat catching one of its sponsons in a wave, while the other sponson clears it. This will cause the boat to *hook*, similar in concept to a jack-knifed truck. Often the boat will *hook* with such force that it stops facing the wrong way on a course.

The fourth type of accident is the *spin out*. This may involve a *hook* or not. Essentially, the boat will catch a wave wrong and suddenly *spin out* of control. An experienced team can drive out of a *spin*, but not without giving the spectators a heart-stopping sight.

The fifth kind of accident is a *fire*. Several different mechanical problems can cause a fire, and it is one of the most discouraging accidents. Since some of the boats are built out of composites, they tend to burn fast, and sink quickly. It is always a tragedy for a team to loose a boat this way, watching their million dollar race craft turn to ashes as they float helplessly in the water.

The *collision* is the sixth type of accident, and is surprisingly rare in offshore racing. The last known collision between two Class I competitors occurred when *Achilli Motors* ran into the side of *Iceberg* at the '91 World Championships. An unfortunate *spin-out* of *Victory 43* in 1993, however, did lead to a collision with a boat of officials.

The final type of offshore accident is the most feared and most common; the *stuff*. In a *stuff* a boat launches off one wave and actually plows through or *stuffs* into the next one. A wave of water will then smash over the bow of the boat, crashing straight into the cockpit. Although some *stuffs* are minor, and only involve the team getting wet, others are harrowing. If a boat goes into a *stuff* at a high enough rate of speed they will actually continue traveling for several boat lengths under water. When this occurs the *stuffing* is called a *submarine*, because that's what the boat resembles when the accident is witnessed from the air. For the paramedics, it is a heart-stopping moment, as they watch and wait for the boat to return to the surface.

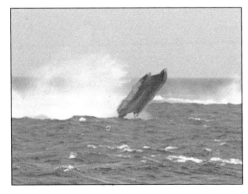 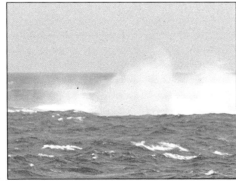 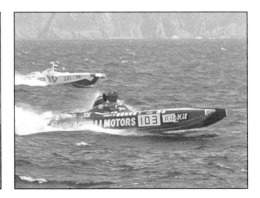

Domenico Achilli's Achilli Motors illustrates a kite. The team drove out of it, but not without jarring themselves hard into their seats.

Photo by D. LLOYD

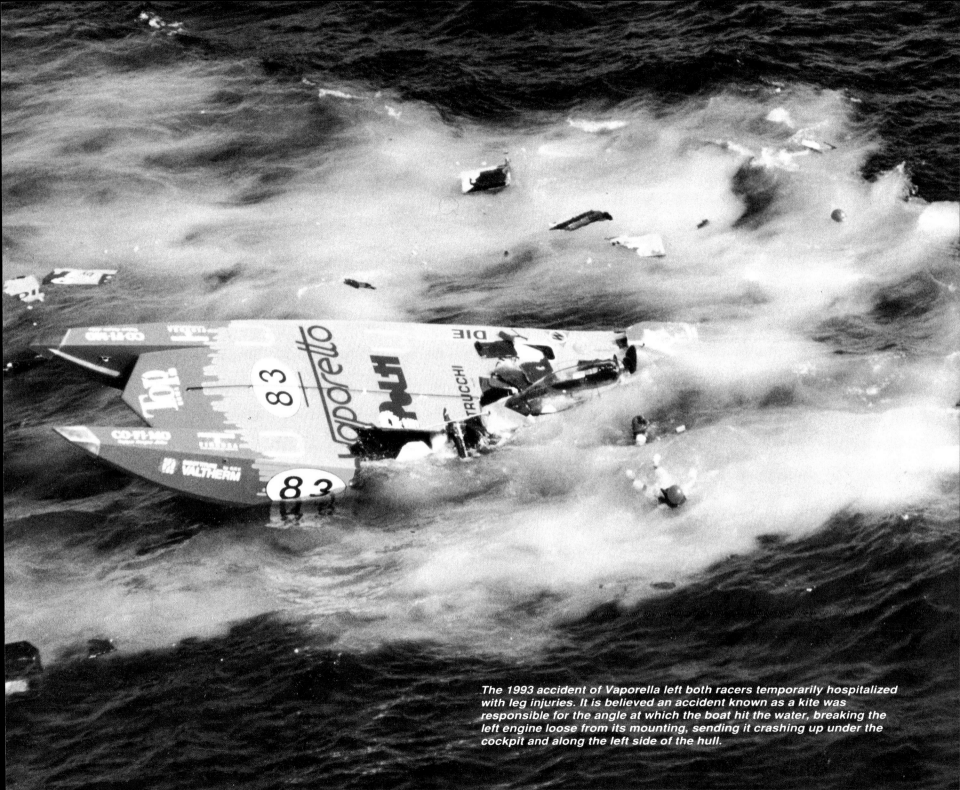

The 1993 accident of *Vaporella* left both racers temporarily hospitalized with leg injuries. It is believed an accident known as a kite was responsible for the angle at which the boat hit the water, breaking the left engine loose from its mounting, sending it crashing up under the cockpit and along the left side of the hull.

Studies Lead to Safety

It was from the study of these seven types of accidents that current safety measures have been incorporated into boat racing. Perhaps the most important is the adaptation of the canopy into the hull design of the boat.

The canopy is the clear, protective shell covering the drivers as they sit in the cockpit. Originally modeled after the F-16 fighter plane canopy, canopies now come in a variety of different shapes and sizes.

The first canopy was designed by George Linder and appeared on the U.S. Superboat, *The Jesse James*. Although active in the drawings for the boat, owner/driver Mark Lavin perished in a stuffing accident before his new canopied boat was finished. Left to race without his beloved brother, Chris Lavin went on to create the Mark Lavin Safety Foundation, considered experts in the world of offshore safety.

Headed by U.S. physician, Doctor Matt Houghton, the Lavin Safety Foundation was instrumental in pushing the canopy concept into the UIM rule book. It was through their studies to help competitors survive accidents that over 30 racers are still alive today after experiencing accidents that would have been fatal only four years ago.

Dr. Houghton explains:

"In studies of racing accidents prior to use of the canopy system, 70% involved injuries sustained while within the cockpit;

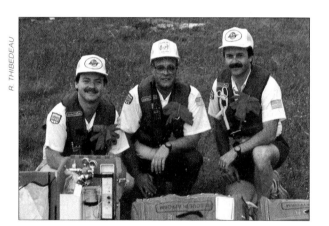

EMT-P David Grattopp, Dr. Matt Houghton, and Dr. Craig Dunham of the Mark Lavin Memorial Safety Foundation.

injuries such as broken ribs or arms suffered when racers bang up against the dash or steering wheel, 20% involve injuries occurring when the racer is ejected from the boat and 10% are water impact injuries either from 'free-flight' water entry or injuries occurring when water crashes into the boat while the racer is still inside. Obviously the water impact injuries are the most dangerous, and the most fatal.

"By moving into canopies with correct seat restraints, circumferential competitor protection and adequate rescue capabilities, the racer actually reduces his chance of injury by 90%, with the only remaining potential injury factor (of those listed) being water impact injuries when water rushes into the open canopy or cracked hull."

Sudden deceleration is the actual cause of injury and death in most stuffing accidents. By meeting a solid wall of water, the boat and the crew are stopped so quickly that many suffer head and neck injuries. By utilizing the new five point harness system, which straps the racers to the seat from belts at both sides of the waist, between the legs, and over each shoulder, the racer isn't as likely to be tossed around inside the cockpit.

By utilizing the correct helmet and canopies, head and neck injuries have been greatly reduced since water that once smashed directly into a race team is now forced up and over the cockpit by the canopy.

Two types of canopies exist on the Grand Prix, the ERC, or

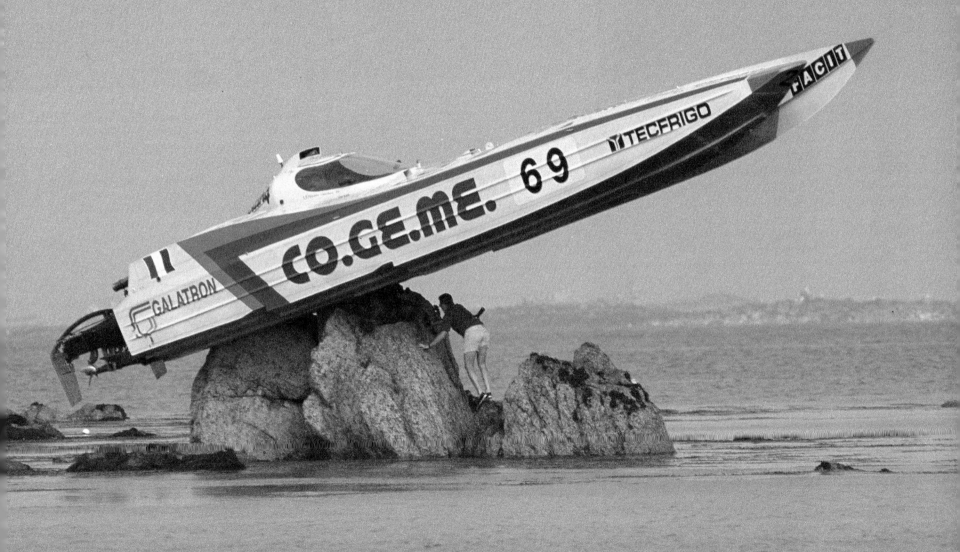

Pansini and Omoboni performed this incredible balancing act with their boat Cogeme while testing in the shallow waters near the wet pits at Guernsey 1993. Although the photograph looks spectacular, Cogeme was logged on the rocks while idling into the pits at high tide, and found balanced in the "trophy" position once the tide went down. PHOTO BY CHRIS DAVIES/PPL

enclosed, reinforced restrained cockpit, and the RRC, or reinforced restrained cockpit. The difference is in the top of the canopy. The ERC has a hatch over the top of it, completely enclosing the racer in the canopy bubble, and the RRC has a hatchless opening at the top, large enough for the racer to move in and out.

Whichever type of canopy a team selects, the most important safety factor is still the competitors themselves. Those racing on the Grand Prix must pass both a pre-season physical, a dunk test and prior to each event, a pre-race physical.

At the end of each race season, and at the first race of each year, the Lavin Foundation and the UIM perform a series of dunk testing, or turtle tests.

In these tests, each racer is strapped into a dunk tester outfitted with a five point harness system. The racer wears his helmet and life jacket. He is strapped into a seat on the "dunker", shaken off balance and then dunked upside down into a swimming pool. The racer is then timed on his ability to release himself from the seat, and how he swims to the surface. Depending upon where he sits in his race boat, the racer will have to swim to the surface on the left or the right of the dunker. If he emerges at the front or back of the dunker he has to take the test again. The purpose of the dunk test is to familiarize the racer with the experience of being upside down and strapped in a seat under

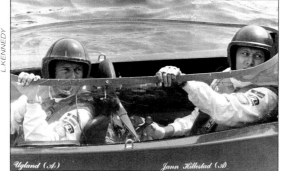

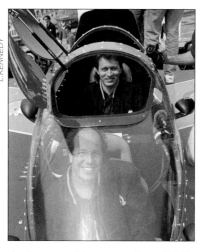

Andreas and Jann race in an RRC - open canopy on their Class III boat, Baby Uno, and in an ERC - enclosed canopy on their Class I boat, BP Valentino.

water. Few racers will say they enjoy dunk testing, but they all recognize that the knowledge learned has helped save lives.

In addition to the canopy and restraint system, several other safety measures are involved in offshore racing. The incorporation of a below deck water deflection, or cage, built around the team protects them from water impact on the side and back as well as the front. This step is built into the boat's construction.

Secondly, each team is responsible for insuring they're familiar with the safety teams at each race. The medical rescue team is on hand throughout the race and preceding testing, and attends all driver's briefings. During the race the medical crew will have stations on land, out in rescue boats and in rescue helicopters. Thorough training of the local teams insures that they can reach an accident site within the first few minutes of an incident.

This coordination of medical crews is a serious challenge to the Grand Prix, especially when considering the many different countries it visits each season. In most rescue boats, for example, at least one multi-lingual person is on hand as a paramedic or translator. Teams must also be given directions to the hospitals at the drivers briefings prior to each race so that their crew and family can locate them if they are taken into emergency.

In the event that a competitor has problems

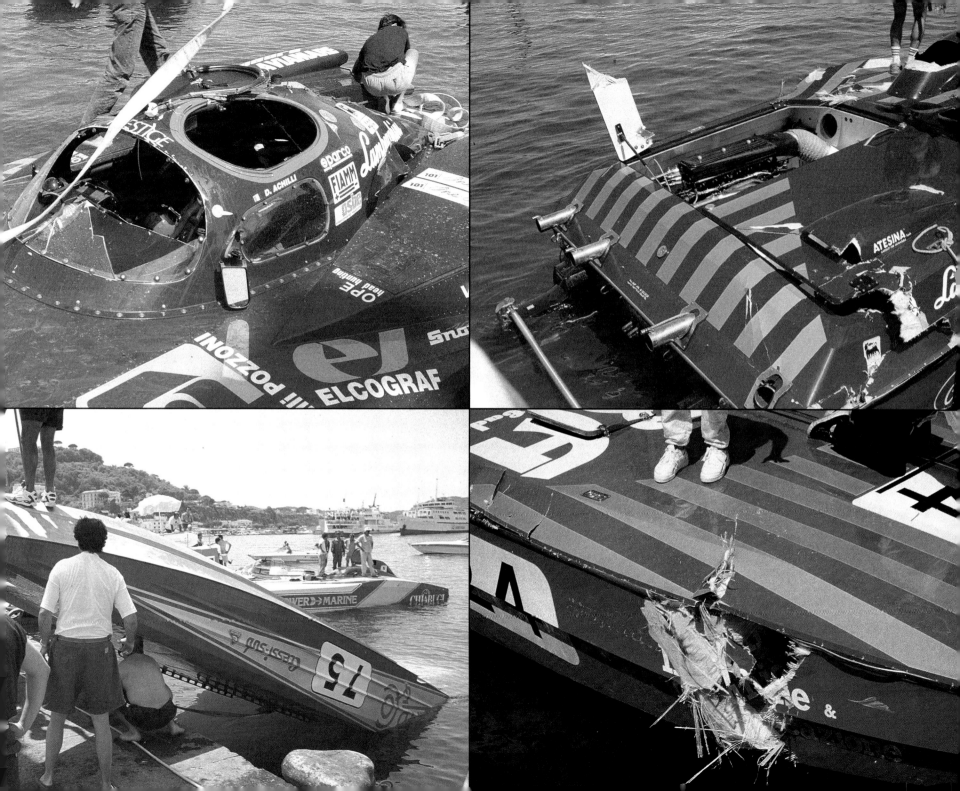

evacuating from an overturned boat, safety rules require each racer to carry airtanks which allow them to breath underwater. These tanks are only necessary if a racer panics or has difficulty getting out of their boat. Further safety equipment includes flares, shark repellent, a device to break open the canopy from the inside, and a knife, strapped to the leg on the outside of their uniform in case the racer has to cut themselves out of their restraint system.

Special safety devices involved in offshore racing include the "kill switch". This is necessary should one of the two racers loose consciousness and their co-driver needs to shut off the boat. Attaching the "kill switch" via a cord to a racer's arm ensures that the boat will shut off after an accident as well, making it safer for paramedics to approach a disabled boat.

Even the rescue equipment itself has evolved over the years. New to offshore racing since the inception of the canopy are smaller, lightweight life-vests, important for teams moving in and out of canopied cockpits. For the paramedics there is the new inflatable stretcher which inflates in water, lifting the injured racer to the surface in a prone position. It has built in handles, making it easier to move a racer from the water onto

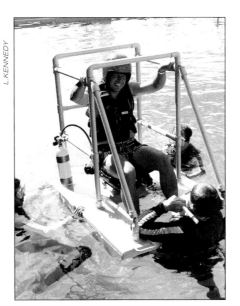

Andreas Ugland steadies himself to be turned over in the dunk test.

a medic boat or nearby race boat.

Finally, the UIM rules stipulate that the first team to arrive on the scene of an accident must stop to render assistance until medical crews arrive. Many a fellow racer has aborted a race and dived into the sea to help another team evacuate from their boat. To insure that a leading team doesn't loose points when this occurs, the UIM rules guarantee that no matter what position a team is running in at the time they stop to render assistance in an accident they are awarded that position and points at the end of the day, whether they finish or not.

Racers who have survived accidents have expressed great satisfaction with the UIM safety procedures, especially the dunk test. The worse thing experienced in an accident is the act of being turned upside down in dark, cold water. Disorientation can cause a racer to swim up inside the hull of the boat, back towards the engines or cause them to swim the entire length of the boat instead of taking a quick exit to the side. By incorporating canopies and five point harness systems, testing in the dunk tester, and building stronger boats, more and more racers are not only surviving accidents, but coming out strong enough and smart enough to race again another day.

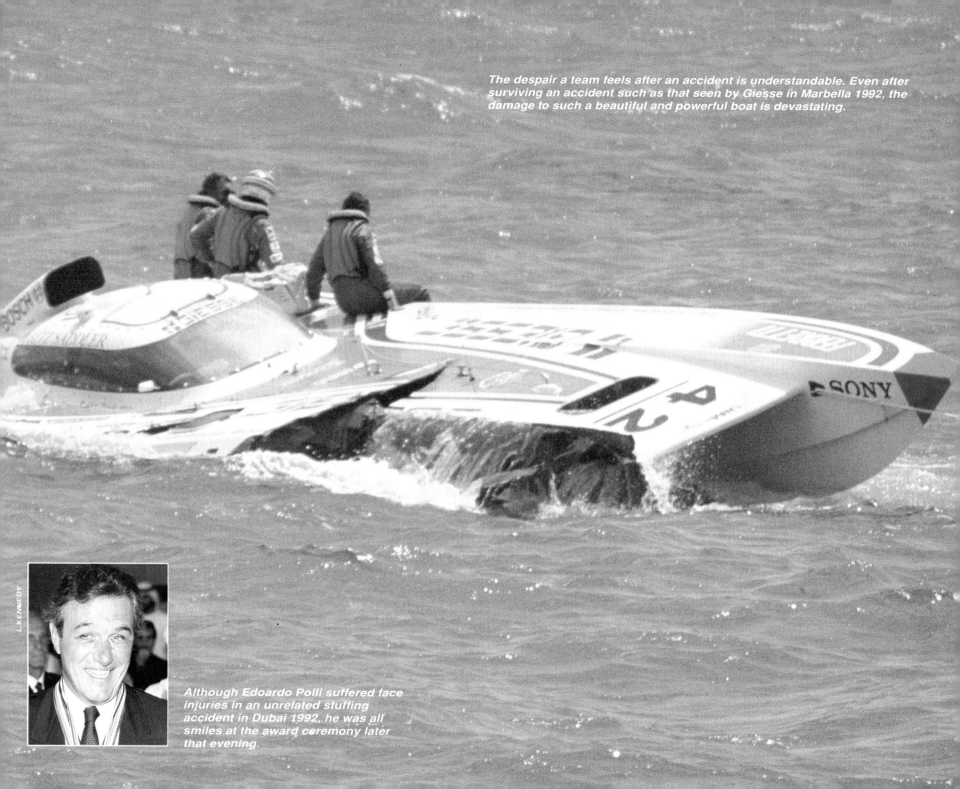

The despair a team feels after an accident is understandable. Even after surviving an accident such as that seen by Giesse in Marbella 1992, the damage to such a beautiful and powerful boat is devastating.

L.KENNEDY

Although Edoardo Polli suffered face injuries in an unrelated stuffing accident in Dubai 1992, he was all smiles at the award ceremony later that evening.

Chapter 6
Winning is Everything

Every team on the Offshore Grand Prix has at some time developed the grace to accept defeat with dignity. Yet each will gladly admit they'd much rather be on the winner's podium than in the adoring crowd.

In offshore racing winning is everything. As the technology grows in offshore, so too does the expense. Winning not only means a team can enjoy a moment in the limelight, but it's that very limelight that enables them to get and keep a sponsor. And without a sponsor, few teams can afford to race.

Perhaps that's why the winner's podium is such an exuberant place. Many of the racers are previous winners, not only in offshore, but in most every sport they tackle. Steven Curtis, at only 30 years old, is a two time World Champion and the 1992 Pole Position Champion. Andreas and Jann have been Class III World Champions twice, and 1990 Class II European Champions. Kjell Rokke and Jim Dyke have been U.S. National Champions and OPT World Champions. Randy Scism and Hamad Buheleba have been Middle Eastern Champions twice. Edoardo Polli, Angelo Spelta, Walter Rigazzi and Fabio Buzzi have all seen their fair share of European, Italian and World Championship titles. Yet, come race day, none of those previous titles mean as much as the win that day.

Trophies To Treasure

Ravenna and the local race organizers have historically done a wonderful job at rewarding the winners of a race. There isn't just one awards ceremony, there are two, with a level of world class trophies, medallions, silver and gold cups that keeps on improving in quality.

The greatest improvement in trophies came when the Grand Prix took their final two World Championship races to Dubai, one of the seven United Arab Emirates. The first year the Grand Prix World Champion was determined in Dubai the winners, Walter Rigazzi and J.P. Mattila, took home a gold trophy depicting the skyline of Dubai.

The second year the World Championship was determined in Dubai wonderful trophies were featured as well. Large gold sea shells with a large white "pearl" in the center as well as gold, silver and brass plated medallions for all the competitors. But the most exciting Grand Prix trophies to date were prizes awarded direct from the Maktoum family, the ruling family of Dubai, to the top three teams of 1993. The third place team, *Bilba*, took home a Jaguar motorcar. The second place team, *Giesse*, took home a Mercedes, and the new World Champions, *Victory 4*, took home a Ferrari.

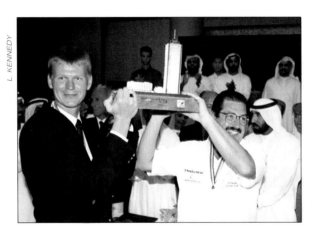
1992 Grand Prix World Champions J.P. Mattilla and Walter Rigazzi took home a gold statue of Dubai with their win.

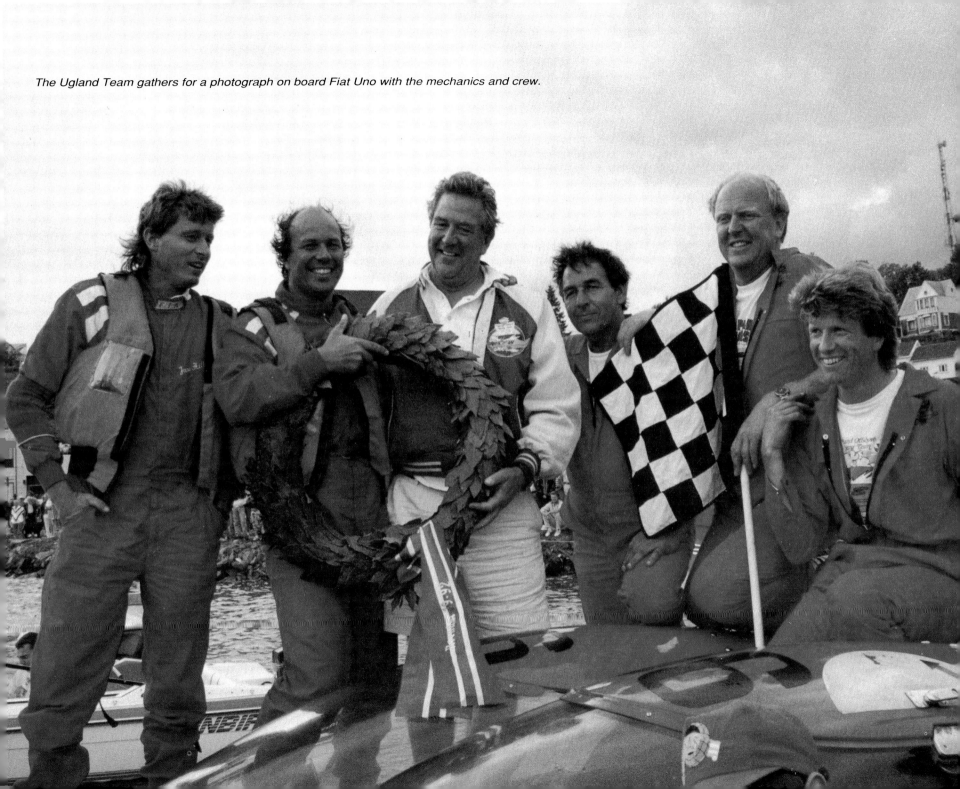

The Ugland Team gathers for a photograph on board Fiat Uno with the mechanics and crew.

The Media

A plus to winning a Grand Prix is the additional media attention a team receives. As the sport has grown in popularity it has attracted media attention from around the globe, in television, magazines and newspapers, movies and radio, as well a number of offshore annuals printed in Europe.

Coverage of an offshore race is more expensive than most motorsports, especially for photographers. The best shots are often taken from the sky, and the sharp shooters who've come to be known as the masters in the craft of offshore photography have become adept at balancing from the edge of a helicopter, stretching out against their safety harness to grab an award winning shot.

Naturally the television cameraman must possess special strength and balance to hold a 30-60 lb camera on his shoulder while balancing himself against the wind. How they manage to deliver consistent steady images is amazing, and the reason

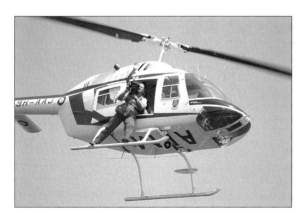

Work for the offshore cameraman involves a balancing act typically seen at the circus.

many local race-site television stations work with these professionals. Not only are they the best, but they are often the only cameramen crazy enough to love doing it.

When the *Victory Team* joined the Grand Prix they brought with them the interest of the Middle East viewing audience. Dubai Television covered the 1993 Grand Prix all season, filming from a variety of different locations on land and in the air, mixing the show during the night and showing it during prime-time viewing hours the next day. Broadcasting to both Arabic and English viewers, Dubai Television's broadcasts featured Thani Juma as the Arabic announcer and Derrick Lloyd commentating in English.

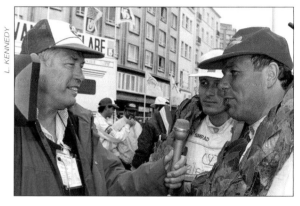

Dubai Television's Derrick Lloyd interviews the Ugland Team after 1993 Belgium Grand Prix.

Once completed, Dubai Television's broadcasts are shown throughout the Middle East, Asia and Australia.

SPES handled organization of the Grand Prix's television coverage with networks and production companies in Italy, France, Belgium and the United Kingdom. These contacts often supply footage for the rest of the world, but as the circuit grows network coverage will include the United States, Scotland, Norway and other countries as well.

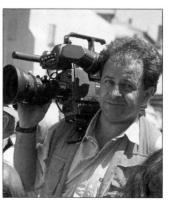

SPES cameramen cover the events from land and air.

No one gets closer to offshore than the helicopters, as the larger photo will illustrate. Very few helicopters are allowed to fly over a race's protected air space, the only aircraft allowed carry medics, camera crews and race organizers. Inger Ugland (bottom right) enjoys the jump seat next to the pilot, the only seat open to guests, family and VIPs.

Photos by L. KENNEDY

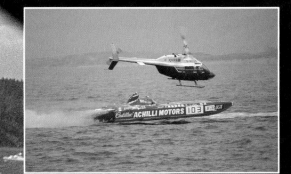

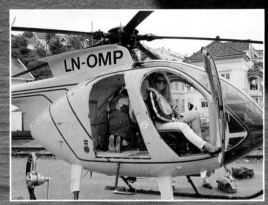

Television coverage is also generated by several different groups of independent film companies doing documentaries on the sport. The Production Company of Jersey, England, for example, produced a show called *Fast Boats, Hard Water* in 1990, which covered the danger and safety of racing and was still seeing air time three years later. Other companies such as FM Television, and Georgio Vascena also produce documentaries on individual teams and race sites, some of which are used for television programing, others to generate sponsorship for teams and race sites.

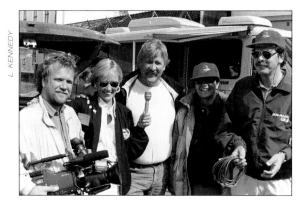

Vascena (far right) utilizes his Italian production crew and those from host countries and other companies filming as well.

Independents are a big source of coverage in offshore, and no where is that more evident than in the circle of freelance photographers. Photographic agencies such as Sea & See Italia send their top sports photographers to cover offshore. Talents like Carlo Borlenghi and Glen Philip Hagen catch the sport on film and wire it throughout the world. Other freelancers like Franco Bartolini and Mario Brenna cover the marine publishing industry, often working directly for some of the world's best magazines. Their on-the-spot coverage has provided some of the most captivating memories of the sport - boats frozen in mid-flight after launching off a wave, teams swimming to the surface after surviving an accident, water smashing over a cockpit, crowds surging to reach a racer - memories which are circulated via the print media and in offshore annuals.

Freelance writers are also a force in carrying information on the Grand Prix around the world. Some work for teams as public relations professionals and supplement their income by writing race coverage for magazines and newspapers. Others work directly for national magazines and newspapers, writers such as John Walker, Ray Bulman, and Dag Pike. These writers often have filed away race coverage that goes back several years, eventually becoming a good source for information on the history of the sport as well.

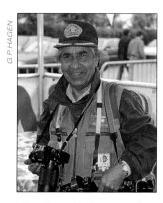

Re Fraschini covers the action from land or sea.

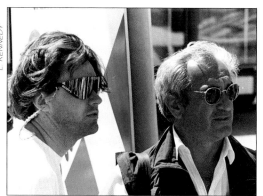

Photographers Glenn Philip Hagen and Carlo Borlenghi.

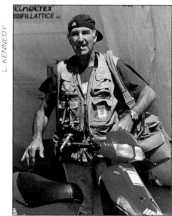

Photographer Franco Bartolini carries his bag of tricks.

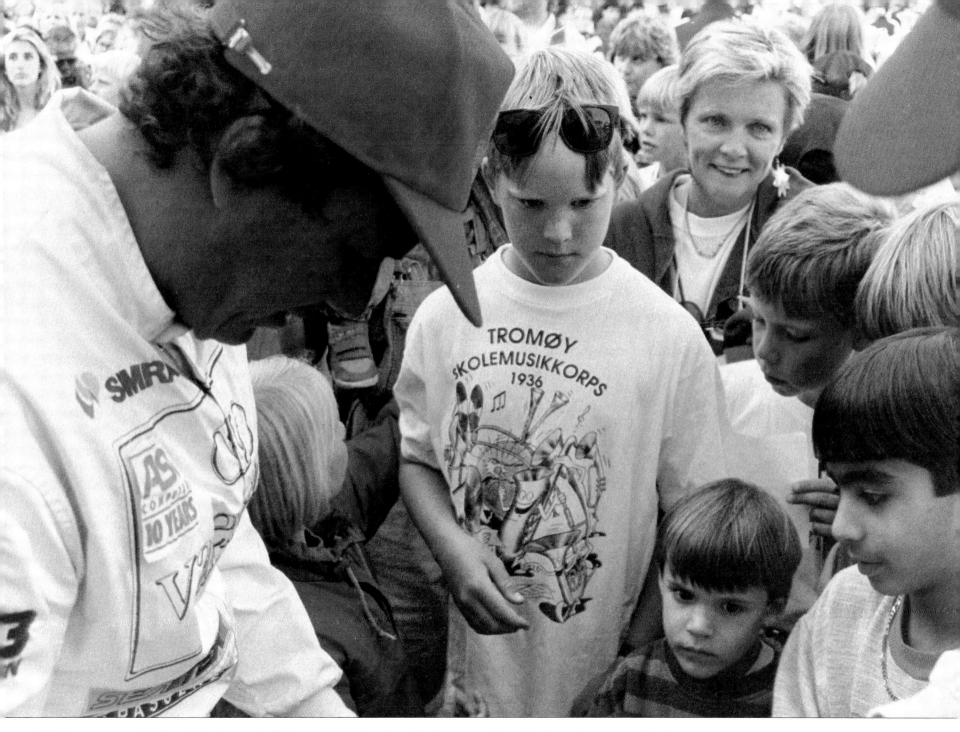

Children are especially fond of the heros of offshore, which is just fine with the racers who make themselves accessible for autographs and photographs after a race.

The Crowds

More and more people have become fans of offshore racing, and the numbers keep growing as the Grand Prix travels all throughout Europe. In 1993 alone it appeared in Spain, Italy (twice), France, England, Belgium and Dubai. Racers from the Grand Prix also were involved in offshore events on series within their own countries, as well as the European Championship and endurance racing. Approximately 20 different events were carried out in Europe between the months of May and November, each of them drawing thousands of spectators to the pits, and anywhere from 50-250 thousand on race day.

The Grand Prix, as all offshore racing, offers free spectator viewing. That, and the fact that organizers design their courses for maximum visibility along the most popular beachfronts, makes the Grand Prix accessible to everyone. Fans of offshore can enjoy a race from a spectator boat at sea, while enjoying a picnic with their family on the beach, or while sitting in the comfort of their beachfront balcony.

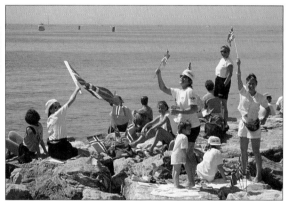

Hours before the race in Marbella, Spain, Norwegian fans claimed their spot on the rocks to cheer for Kjell Rokke's Brooks Shoes.

Some sites plan special race day activities, such as in Dubai where the Corniche hosts over 150,000 locals to a day of offshore racing and beachfront entertainment. Food vendors, first aid stations and personal facilities are set up along the beach next to bleachers and a professional sound stage. Spectators show up early in the morning to enjoy the music and dancing before the race, then it's all eyes on the sea as the Grand Prix begins.

In Valetta, Malta, spectators line the rocks and monuments along the shoreline. In Arendal, Norway it's the fjords that fill with race fans from early morning. In Guernsey, the spectator fleet is so large that when viewed from a distance it looks like an island itself.

Most race sites also set aside a special viewing area for race volunteers, crew and family members - people who would need to get back to the wet pits in a hurry should there be an emergency or a rush to be with their family at the winners circle. These areas are usually adjacent to the pits.

On the whole, the sea front belongs to the spectators, and they show their appreciation with consistent spectator attendance unlike that enjoyed by any other sport in the world.

Facing Page - The crowds come out for offshore!
Top Left: Arendal, Norway. Top Right: Valletta, Malta
Bottom Left: Poole, England. Bottom Right: Dubai, U.A.E.
Poole photo by L. KENNEDY, Balance by D. LLOYD

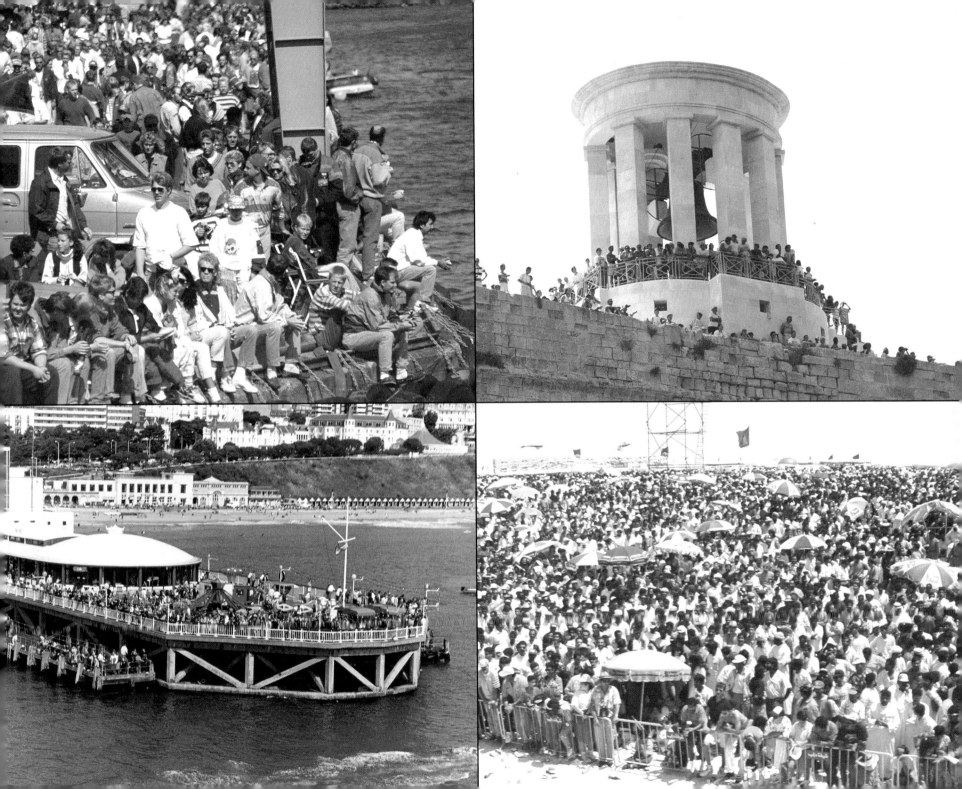

L. KENNEDY

The Celebration

Little needs to be said about the photographs on the next few pages. They are as much a part of The Grand Prix as anything else. The race is over, the victory won, and now the teams are allowed to celebrate.

Laurel wreaths, champagne and trophies are a big part of winning, but so are the smiles shared with friends and family. The most enjoyable winner's podiums occur when one of the winning teams has taken awhile to get there. These celebrations are the best - enthusiasm is high and contagious, not only for the

D. LLOYD

crowd but also for the other teams as well.

So when it's time for celebrations, let the champagne pour, the cheers go up, and the smiles beam on, for tomorrow is another day, another race, another season when the team has to get out there and try all over again.

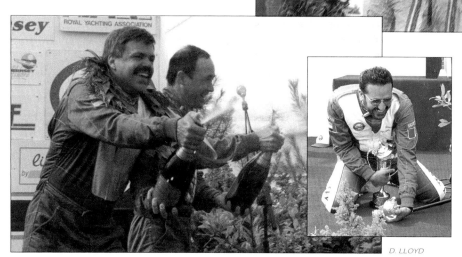

D. LLOYD

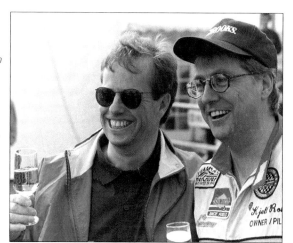

Top, Center and Bottom Right: Spraying the crowd and each other with champagne is a racing tradition. One which Saeed Al Tayer, (Bottom Center) tried to crawl out of.
Kjell Rokke, (Bottom Right) prefers sharing his celebratory champagne with friends and business partner Larrs Ugland.

L. KENNEDY

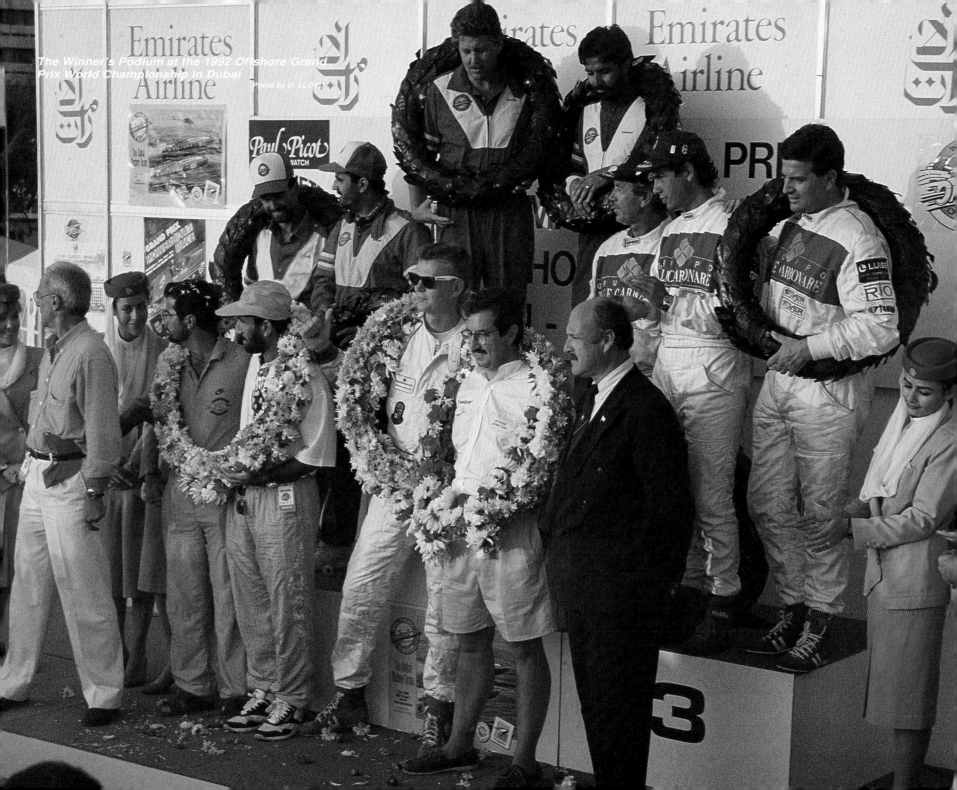

The Winner's Podium at the 1992 Offshore Grand
Prix World Championship in Dubai
Photo by D. LLOYD

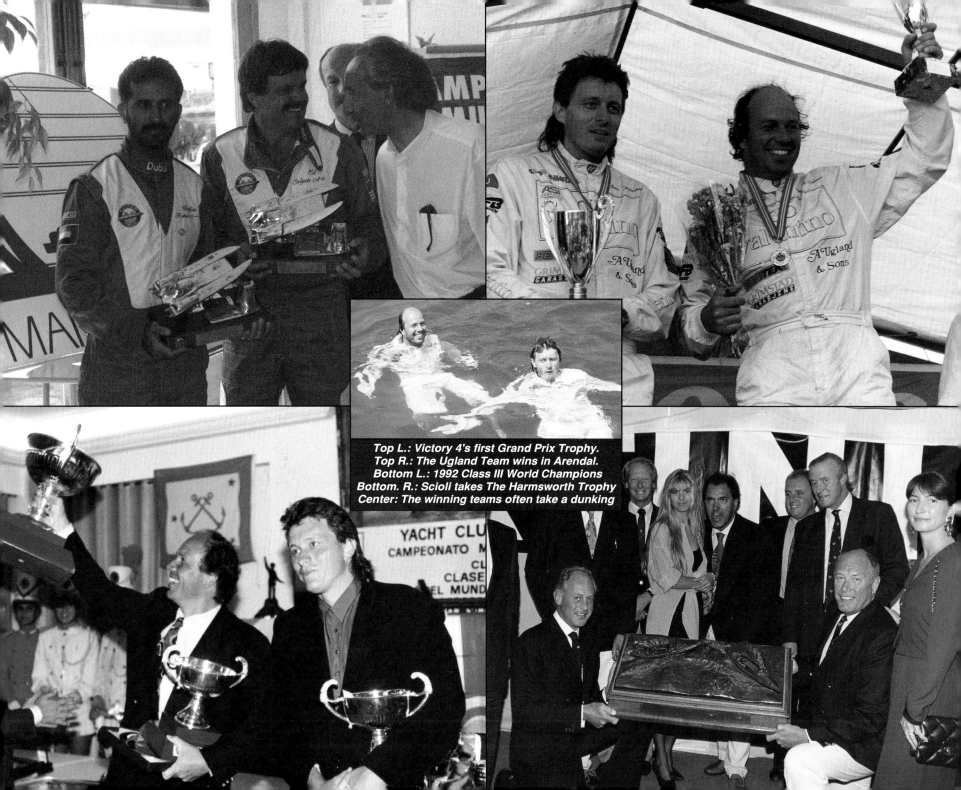

Top L.: Victory 4's first Grand Prix Trophy.
Top R.: The Ugland Team wins in Arendal.
Bottom L.: 1992 Class III World Champions
Bottom. R.: Scioli takes The Harmsworth Trophy
Center: The winning teams often take a dunking

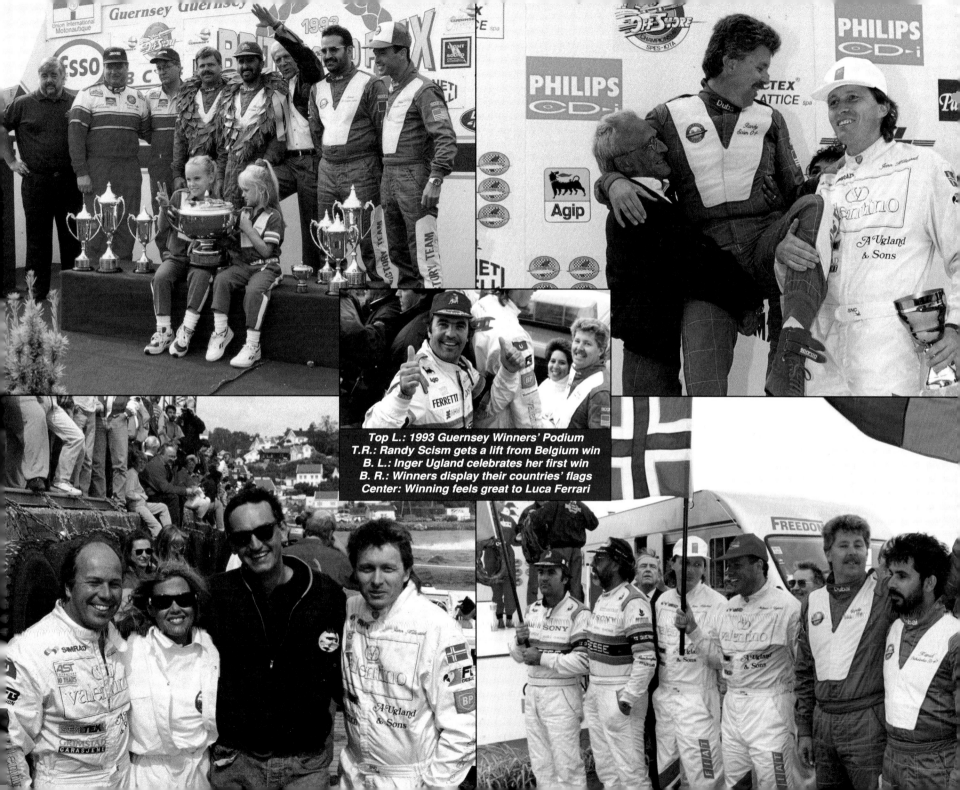

Top L.: 1993 Guernsey Winners' Podium
T.R.: Randy Scism gets a lift from Belgium win
B. L.: Inger Ugland celebrates her first win
B. R.: Winners display their countries' flags
Center: Winning feels great to Luca Ferrari

Chapter 7
Offshore Off Course

Behind the scenes of all the work and preparation a lot of enjoyable times are shared by the teams involved in the Offshore Grand Prix. By traveling to races every two or three weeks over seven months, the offshore fraternity becomes a close knit group. They work side-by-side, travel together, and learn to depend on each other - often times to save each other's lives.

The enjoyable times are what brings the racers together. From a simple afternoon in the pits discussing each other's boats, to an anxiety filled afternoon waiting together at an airport, to a laugh shared at a sponsor party or dinner, the offshore racers cross cultural and language barriers as they learn to compete against their new found friends.

Not every race team, of course, relates closely with everyone else. The group is too big to expect that, yet for the hundred or more people involved, communication exists throughout and there isn't one racer who wouldn't help his fellow competitor if he needed him.

A wide variety of activities go on throughout the year which add to the enjoyment of the Offshore Grand Prix. Boat parades, parties, sponsor engagements and the simple day-to-day work around the pits offer a host of opportunities for race teams and officials to get together. Sharing the same interests makes it easy for friendships to start.

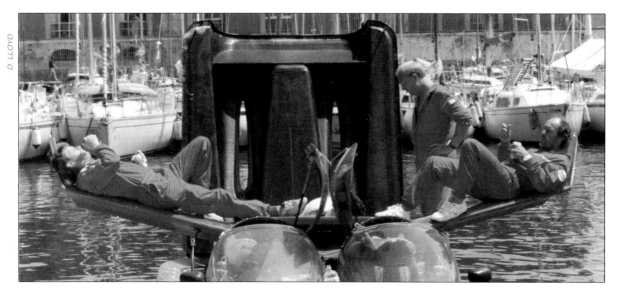

D. LLOYD

Jann and Andreas take a Diet Coke break between legs of an endurance race in 1992.

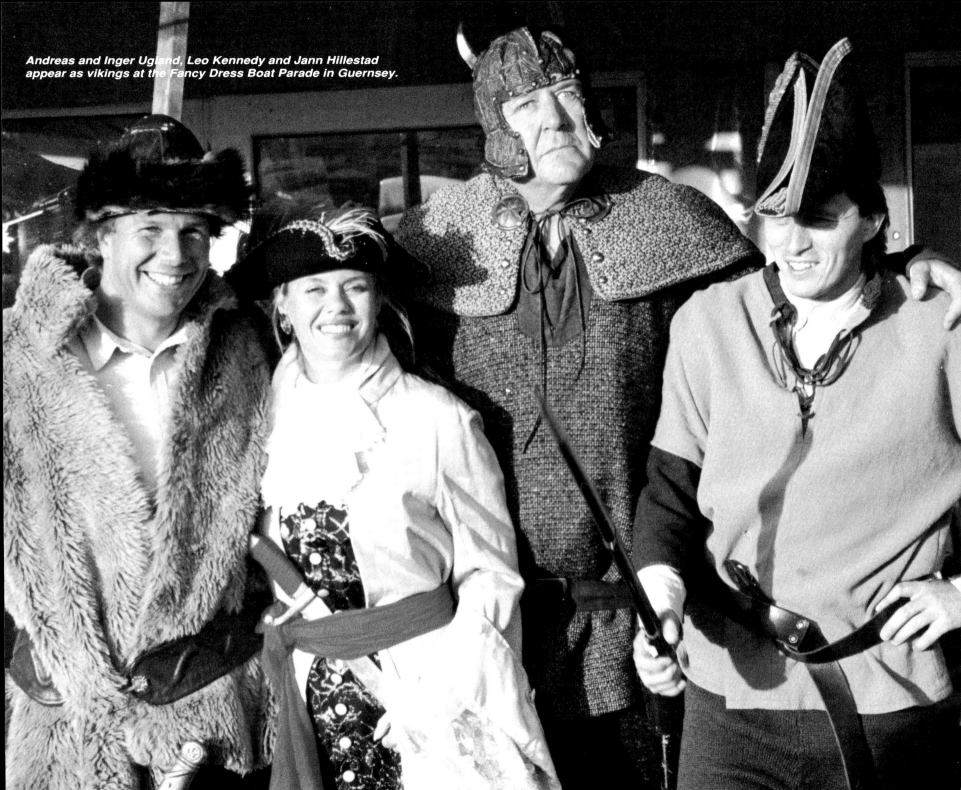

Andreas and Inger Ugland, Leo Kennedy and Jann Hillestad appear as vikings at the Fancy Dress Boat Parade in Guernsey.

Race Time is Family Time

Most racing families are quite close, in fact several teams are made up of fathers and sons racing together with other family members supporting them as pit crew or publicity persons. Other teams consist of brothers, nephews and uncles, husbands and wives or cousins. It seems once the offshore racing bug bites entire families are affected.

Parents often involve their small children in racing in whatever way possible. From washing the boat to running small errands, their children become adept in functioning as valuable members of the team. Other children whose parents aren't racers, such as Offshore Commissioner Richard Ridout's two sons attend most every race of the season and become official junior crew members of teams - helping out whenever they can. The children add a fresh appeal to offshore, especially the smallest

Andreas K. Ugland and his wife attend races throughout the year to support their son's team.

ones who show up at the races decked in their team's uniform, ready to cheer their parent's team on for a big win.

Other family members who become unofficial members of the teams are parents and siblings. Like so many other teams, Andreas' father is active with the team and has attended his events for over eighteen years, and has become a regular member

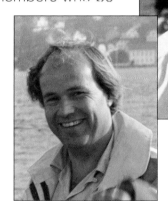

While Johann Ugland (L) has raced himself, Knut Ugland (R) chooses to lend his support to racing by cheering from the shoreline.

of the team. His mother and brothers Knut and Johan attend races whenever possible, their love of competition still evident by their support of Andreas and Jann.

Many racers take great comfort with their family around them, while others need complete concentration before a race and prefer to attend the events alone. Either way, it's the family on site and the family at home who are the first to get the news - news to say the team is okay or to let them know they've won.

L. KENNEDY

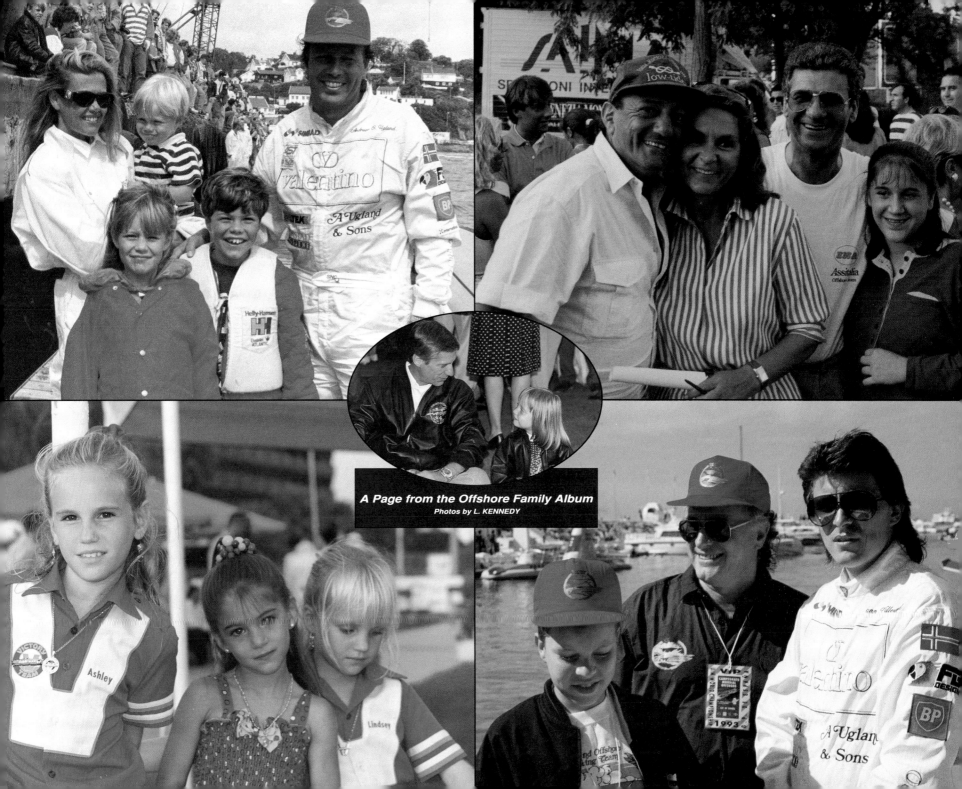

A Page from the Offshore Family Album
Photos by L. KENNEDY

Working with Sponsors

Some sponsors are actively involved in offshore, while others are not. Those that are, seem to not only get a better return on their investment, but more enjoyment as well.

The Ugland Team has worked with a variety of sponsors during the Grand Prix, but the most hands-on sponsor involvement came with their 1993 sponsorship with British Petroleum's Marine Division. Upon signing the sponsorship, BP's offices in England worked with the team and their own advertising agencies to produce a contest published in Sea Trade Magazine where the winners (one from the States, one from Europe) won an all expense paid trip to the Belgium Grand Prix. This was especially enjoyable for Andreas and Jann because the contest winners had never been to an offshore race, or ever seen an offshore boat

up close. Their attendance at the race fueled the emotions of the team, giving them an even greater determination to win. *BP Valentino* lead the event up until breaking a trim tab, and even then had enough of a lead built up that they managed to finish the final two laps at much slower speeds and still take third place.

BP, The Ugland Group and HUAL, all sponsors of the team, conducted corporate meetings during the World Championship in Dubai - meetings which included visits to the pits to meet the team and an afternoon watching the race. This kind of involvement served to inspire the team as well as benefit the sponsor.

Most every team and race site needs the help of sponsors in order to compete at Grand Prix level. The Grand Prix itself has sponsors. Collectively the teams, sites and organizers work diligently to insure that the interests of the sponsors are protected and supported.

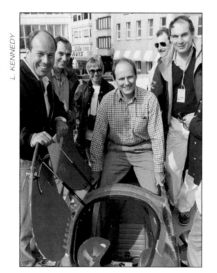

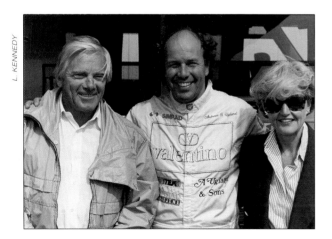

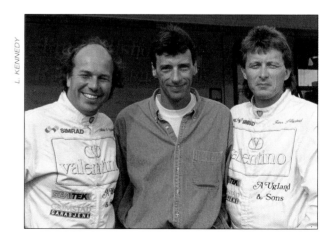

Left: Peter Bertelson, Andreas Ugland and Pru Bertelson of Valentino U.K.
Center: Paul Davis, President of BP Marine and associates gather on top of BP Valentino with Andreas Ugland at the Belguim Grand Prix.
Right: International Paint's Graham Smith joined The Ugland Team for the Guersney Grand Prix.

Special Outings

Every so often an opportunity arises where the teams can participate in special outings that they may otherwise have never enjoyed had it not been for boat racing. These often occur during the World Championships and events where there are several days between races.

In 1991, the Italian Air Force's Exhibition Team, the Frecce Tricolori, invited fifteen racers and support teams out for a visit to the flight deck. The Italian Air Force pilots were as in awe of the offshore

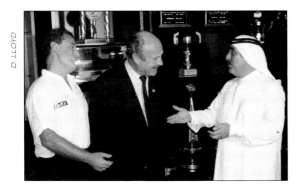

The Frecce Tricolori hosts a group of offshore racers and crew to a visit to their flight deck outside Trieste, Italy.

The *Victory Team* hosts several activities for the teams while they are in Dubai, including open house visitation of the team's headquarters and a party at Sheikh Mana's fish camp.

Other activities enjoyed are golf outings, trips to the desert and falconry, events privately arranged by friends from the *Victory Team* or by the World Championship organizers. One particularly enjoyable outing came when Hamad Buheleba, driver for *Victory #47*, hosted

boats as the offshore pilots were of the tremendous speed and maneuverability of the Frecce Tricolori's F-16s.

a group of racers to his camel ranch in the desert for an evening of camel riding and learning Arab culture.

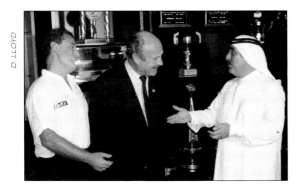
Domenico Achilli and Ralph Fröhling meet with Sheikh Mana at the Victory Team's headquarters.

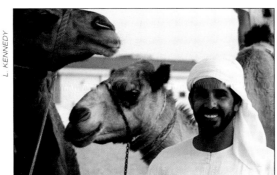
Hamad Buheleba of the Victory Team hosts racers to an evening at his camel ranch.

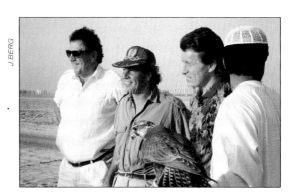
Leo Kennedy, Andreas Ugland and Jann Hillestad learn the ancient sport of falconry.

Getting Around The Races

Just getting to a race can be a challenge for a team. Airlines don't always schedule flights that fit into a team's business plans, so charter planes and helicopters may have to be called in for last minute assistance.

Once on-site, however, getting around the race is another thing altogether. Some dry pits can be over a mile long after the twenty or more teams are lined up one behind another. Competitors and crew also need to travel back and forth to hotels, driver's meetings and other functions as well. Teams learn early that they need compact methods of transportation around the pits.

Custom painted bicycles, scooters, and mopeds, make up the majority of the transportation choices. Other teams avoid the streets, taking a short cut across the water via water taxis, rubber dinghies and small boats. The most unusual transportation mode is used by Jann Hillestad who enjoys getting around the pits on a unicycle. Fast? No...but it's easy to park and he enjoys it when people stand back and clear the way.

Kjell Rokke's *Brook's Shoes* Corvette is the most luxurious mode of race site transportation, but it only seats two. For larger crowds he's been known to incorporate his 40+ foot camper as a makeshift bus.

The *Victory Team* has always made a strong impression, this time in their small fleet of Harley Davidson Motorcycles.

Other specialty items, such as tandem bicycles and micro-scooters, electric skate boards, antique and luxury cars show up at events closer to a racer's home.

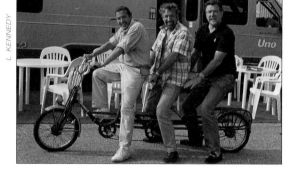

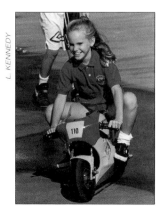

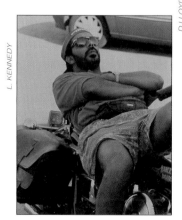

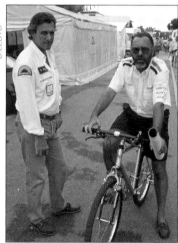

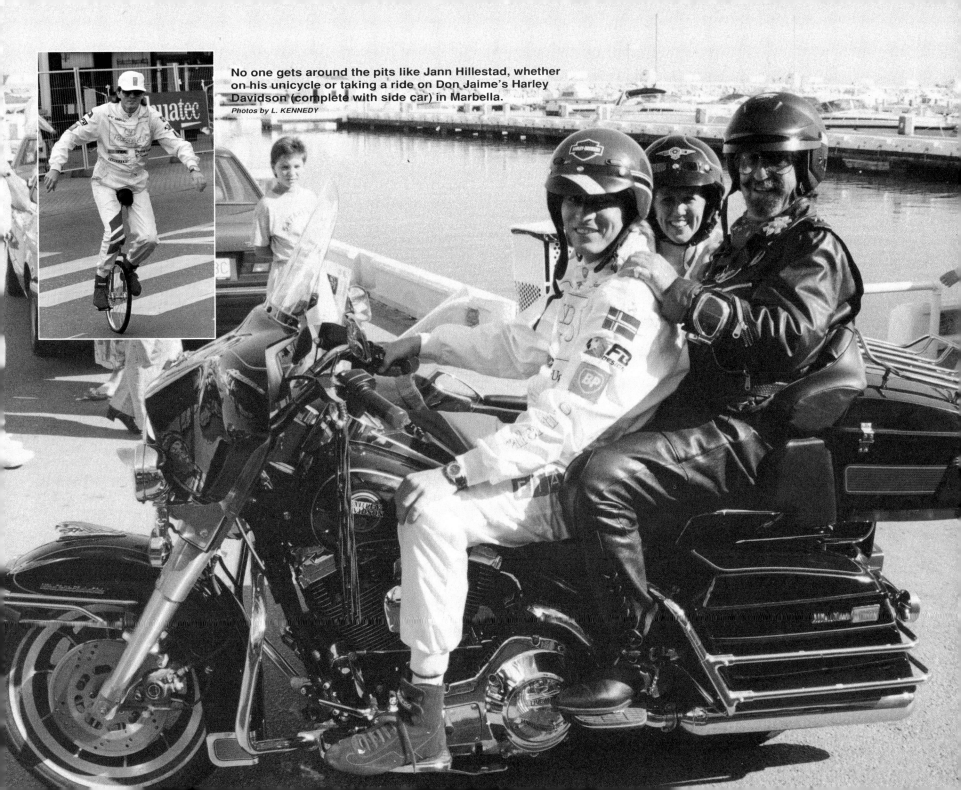

No one gets around the pits like Jann Hillestad, whether on his unicycle or taking a ride on Don Jaime's Harley Davidson (complete with side car) in Marbella.
Photos by L. KENNEDY

The Personalities

It seems every team has its own clown; one member of the crew who's always getting into crazy predicaments and bringing all manners of fun to everyone around them. Several racers are so well known for their friendly outgoing nature that they act as entertainers for the rest of the field. Steve Curtis is known throughout the circuit for his fun-loving, mischievous behavior, as is Richard Carr, Massimo Lippi, Antonio Giofreddi, Dulio Boffi, Hamad Buheleba, and Paulo Patergnani. From the non-racer side Leo Kennedy, David Corsen and Richard Ridout are often found mixing up some sort of creative trouble and lots of fun.

In the midst of the most serious of events, racers often find themselves in predicaments they can't avoid. Saeed Al Tayer, for example, was pulled over by a film crew in Dubai while wearing European shorts and a tee-shirt instead of his customary Arabic dishdash. He quickly borrowed a head-dress for the video taping, thinking he'd solved his problem. Unfortunately the print media began photographing his comical attire while he was on camera and could do nothing to stop them.

A wonderful personality in St. Tropez is local restaurateur Edna Faloau. A Norwegian by birth, Edna welcomes the Grand Prix as an opportunity to host the Norwegian teams to a sumptuous dinner at her

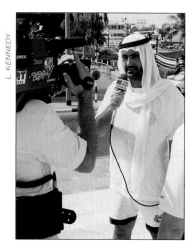

Saeed Al Tayer tries his best to look official in an on-the-spot television interview.

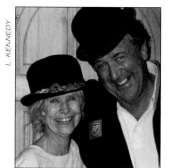

Edna Faloau and Leo Kennedy.

restaurant, closing it down to everyone else in St. Tropez first!

In Puerto Banus/Marbella, the king of the scene is local celebrity Don Jaime, who at 60+ years of age, appears at race site and everywhere else in full black leather astride his Harley Davidson complete with side car.

Personalities from around the globe often appear at races. Film and recording stars, fashion designers, models and public officials all make visits to offshore events. Most fun is when athletes, especially those competing in other motorsports, attend an event. European car racer Will Hoy appeared at the 1992 Guernsey race and jumped into the cockpit with Jann only to return, quite shaken, to the pits some time later.

The ride was a lot rougher than Hoy expected and the notion that he couldn't control the speed had him alarmed. "The pounding the boat takes is quite incredible and the spring-loaded seat was essential," Hoy explained. "Even so, I am convinced that powerboat racers must get shorter with age,"

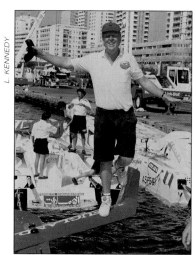

Johannes knows how to balance fun with serious race work.

1991 British Touring Car Champion Will Hoy jumped at the chance to drive
Fiat Uno, but seemed most happy to get out of the boat later!
Photo by L. KENNEDY

The Women

What would any sport be like without the many beautiful women they so often attract? Perhaps it's the sunshine and outdoors, perhaps the lure of the sea, but for some reason the sport of offshore seems to attract more than its fair share of fascinating women, giving the many photographers much more to capture on film than just the race.

Many of the beauties are associated with the event, serving as trophy queens, sponsor hostesses or as part of a team's staff, friends or family. Others are locals taking an afternoon or evening to stroll the pits and enjoy the color and excitement of offshore.

Sporting their team's colors, the women involved in offshore bring style and grace to the sport, supporting and calming the men on their teams, reminding everyone that behind every successful man is a good woman...or two, or three...or ?

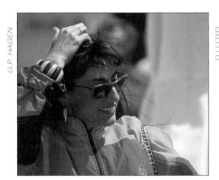
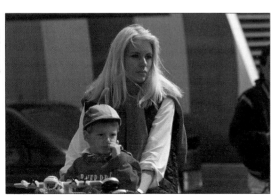
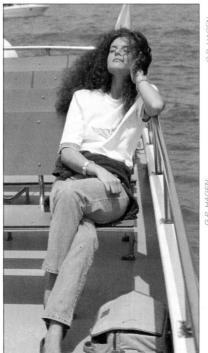
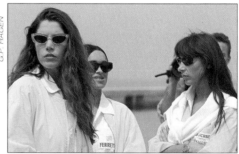
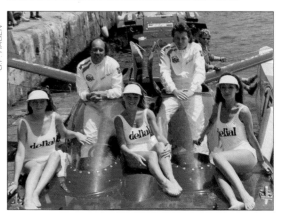

VENEZIA-INTERNAZIONALE OFFSHORE-1992

low-tide

D.LLOYD

Domenico Cirilli may not have won the race, but he was determined to take first prize by walking off with the trophy queen, Miss Italy.

Chapter 8
There's No Turning Back

With eight regular season races scheduled and several European and endurance races on their calendar, the Ugland Team was easily one of the busier teams during the 1993 season. Unbeknownst to the rest of the team, Andreas had his reasons. With his company going public and plans to take over another business, Andreas knew that 1993 may well be his last full season of racing for a while. Though the decision wasn't one he wanted to make, it was one he had to decide on, and one he had to break to Jann.

Jann had, by 1993, raced with Andreas a total of twelve years. The duo had formed a strong friendship which was nurtured by the busy race schedule that drew them from their homes - Jann's in Oslo, Andreas' in London. Cutting back on racing meant Andreas would not be seeing Jann and his many other racing friends as much as he gotten used to.

Jann reflects back on the moment Andreas informed him of his plans to retire:

"Andreas and I were very excited about our new boat BP Valentino after the first 1993 race in Marbella. We believed strongly on our chances in the forthcoming races. Before the Ischia race we had heard Fabio had improved the boat with many more modifications. Tests on the lake in Italy showed an unbelievable speed of more than 135 mph and we were really looking forward to a good race in Ischia.

"Before the Pole Position race in Ischia Andreas and I had a walk around the pit area, talking about different things. We were quite happy with our situation and enjoyed being among the favorites of the race. Suddenly Andreas said: "Jann I must tell you something...This will be our last season on the Grand Prix. I can't continue like this because I am too busy with my work and away from my children too much. I just wanted to say this now, so you can get familiar with my decision during the rest of the season."

"I was quite surprised hearing this from Andreas at that moment, but kept calm and answered: "I understand Andreas, everything must always come to an end, we both know that and I will always remember our time together in the boat as the most exciting and enjoyable moments of my life. Thank you for being so open with me."

"That's what I said to him, but inside I was thinking; Oh no! This can't be true! We are currently running the best boat in the world and the world is laying at our feet. Andreas is talking from his head, not his heart. I know it's even harder for him to quit than for me.

"I tell myself to accept the reality. Whether we like it or not, the sport is taking too much time from our lives and now the time has come to do something about that. To force myself into a better mood I told myself that if we do well in the forthcoming races Andreas will be very excited and realize more and more that it will be impossible for him to quit the sport completely. I decide to support his decision 100% and told myself to only concentrate on and enjoy the upcoming races.

"Then Andreas said: "Jann, you know we can't stay completely out of the sport. We will always be involved in some way. Let's just look at this as a temporary break with at least next year away from the Grand Prix."

"Then I smiled, because through it all I realized that Andreas was thinking exactly the same as I was."

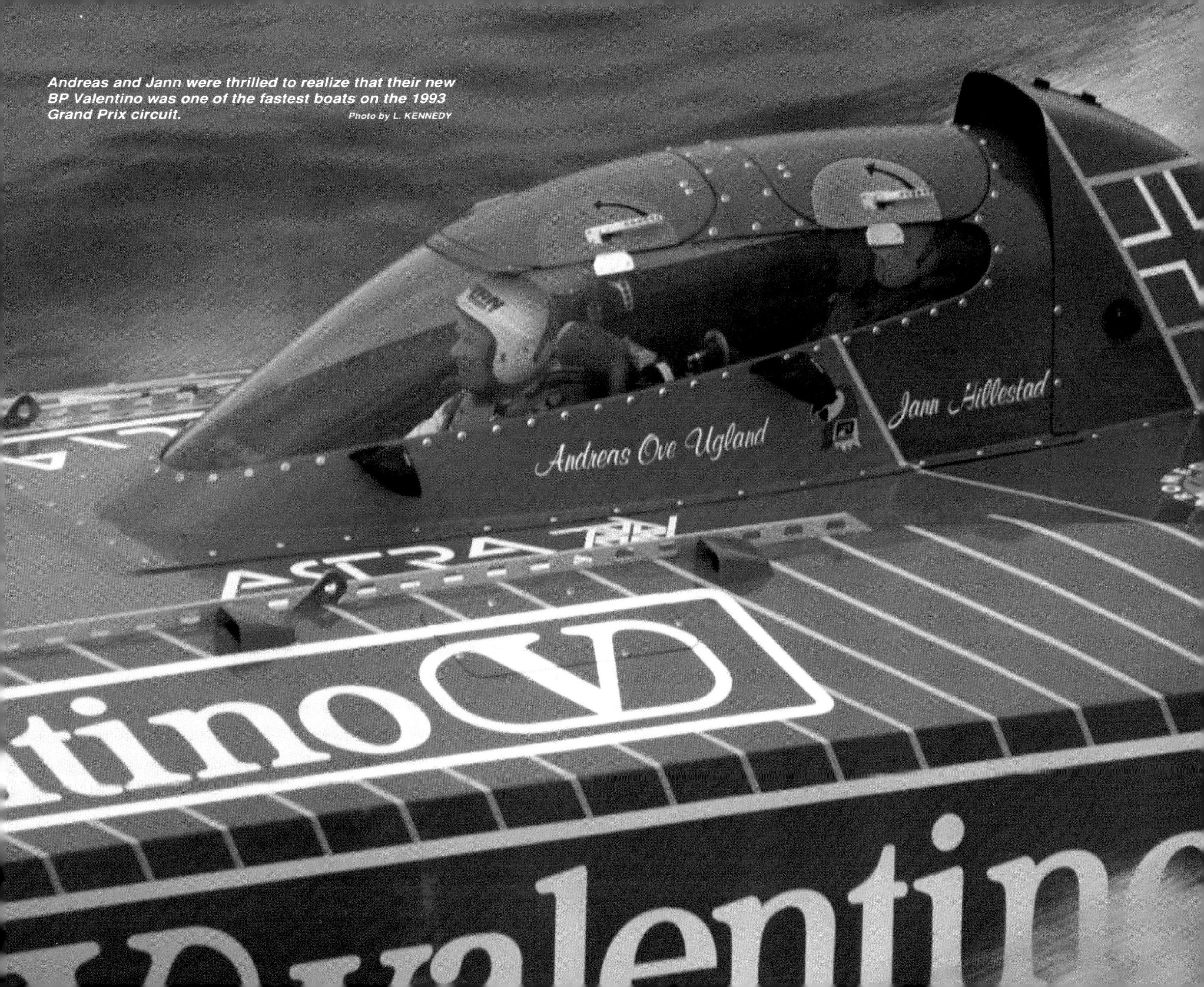

Andreas and Jann were thrilled to realize that their new BP Valentino was one of the fastest boats on the 1993 Grand Prix circuit. Photo by L. KENNEDY

Andreas' decision to take time off from racing for at least a season cast a subtle shadow over the team. Everyone recognized that Andreas didn't really want to retire, so they held out hopes throughout the season that he'd change his mind. Yet, one by one the reminders came in that the decision was serious. During the middle of a light-hearted lunch or dinner Andreas would be approached by teams trying to talk him out of retiring or wanting to purchase *BP Valentino*. Whenever this happened Leo, Gianfranco, Jann and other members of the team would look solemnly at each other. Each and every race became a reminder that the clock was ticking away. The day Andreas announced his sale of the boat to Vincenzo Polli and John Balzarini was the day everyone knew the retirement was for real.

Andreas knew much of what he enjoyed about racing was shared by his team, and that unless the crew found another team, his retirement would affect them as well. Consequently he did what he could to help them find other work and tried his best to make the season as enjoyable as possible for everyone.

Andreas attempted to overload everyone on racing. Racing not only the Grand Prix, but also the European Circuit and

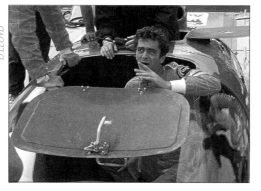

Vincenzo Polli signed the deal to buy the BP Valentino while in Guernsey, 1993.

several endurance races he seemed to think that if he worked them enough they'd be glad for his retirement. Instead everyone had all the more fun and grew even closer.

On the European circuit, the team saw Andreas and Jann take first place finishes in Arendal, Norway and Poole, England. With only two more races scheduled in the Championship, Andreas had to miss the third race, and flew into Trieste for the last leg, only to have the race cancelled due to foul weather. The team took the European Championship for Class I hands down.

Racing in Class III on the European circuit in Arendal, Andreas and Jann managed to win two first place finishes - one in Class I and one in Class III only hours apart, winning their second Class III Championship in-a-row.

Long distance endurance racing made for another avenue the Ugland Team competed in during the 1993 racing season. Returning to the *Fiat Uno* which had been re-rigged as a four passenger endurance boat, Andreas and Jann came in third at the Cowes-Torquay race off the coast of England, a tough but well respected event.

The Ugland Team competed in three different boats in 1993. The Class I BP Valentino catamaran, the Class III Baby Uno, and the Fiat Uno which was used in endurance racing.

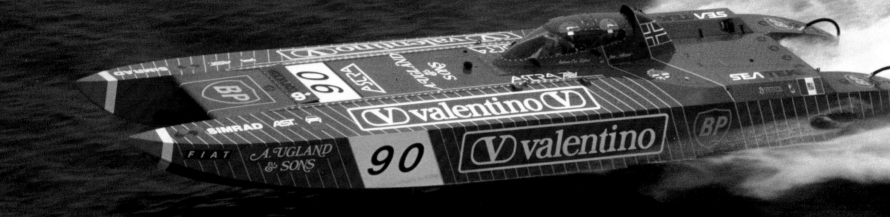

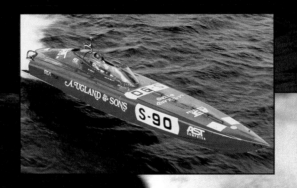

BP Valentino photo by L. Kennedy
Baby Uno photo by G.P. Hagen
Fiat Uno photo by Mario Brenna

Setting The Record Straight

In his contract with Polli and Balzarini, Andreas insured that he did not turn over *BP Valentino* until the first of the new year. This enabled the Ugland Team to make one final attempt at entering the record books in 1993.

On a cold day in December, Andreas and Jann joined Fabio Buzzi and several other teams on Lake Como, Italy for what has come to be an annual event for Europeans striving to break world speed records. With a slight fog covering the lake, Fabio joined Andreas in the cockpit for an attempt at American racer Al Copeland's Class I Speed Record of 138.51 mph set six years earlier in the States.

Starting from the far side of the lake, *BP Valentino* was lost in the fog as it approached the bridge. Running at approximately 100 mph at the point of the first marker buoy, Ugland and Buzzi were in a nine-mph wake zone, doing 91 miles over the limit and sending a rooster tail of water up over the bridge. The local police were soon on the scene to stop "that crazy boat trying to wash cars off the bridge", but it was too late...Andreas and Fabio had already passed the second fixed marker and set a new World Speed Record for Class I - 145.16 mph (233.614 kph).

Jann, who stayed on shore to watch the attempt was anxious to get into the cockpit himself. Together he and Andreas returned to Lake Como to set another record, breaking the current FONDA World Speed Distance Record of 103.49 mph with a new speed of 104.75 mph. The FONDA record was not a kilo attempt, instead it consisted of the average speed held by the boat as it maneuvered a short, 24 mile course.

By the end of the day several records were broken by other teams, but the Class I record was the most impressive, not only for its speed and the 6.65 mph margin over Copeland's record, but because the record had stood for so long. The only recorded speed faster than that set by Andreas Ugland and Fabio Buzzi that day belongs to Hawaiian Tom Gentry who's Superboat World Speed Record of 148.938 was set with a boat carrying almost twice the horsepower as *BP Valentino*.

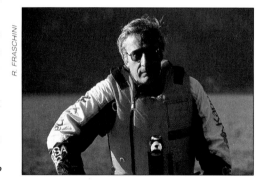

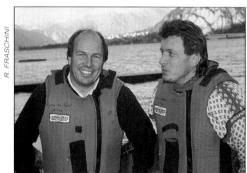

Andreas took two World Speed Records with two different throttlemen, Fabio Buzzi (top) and Jann Hillestad.

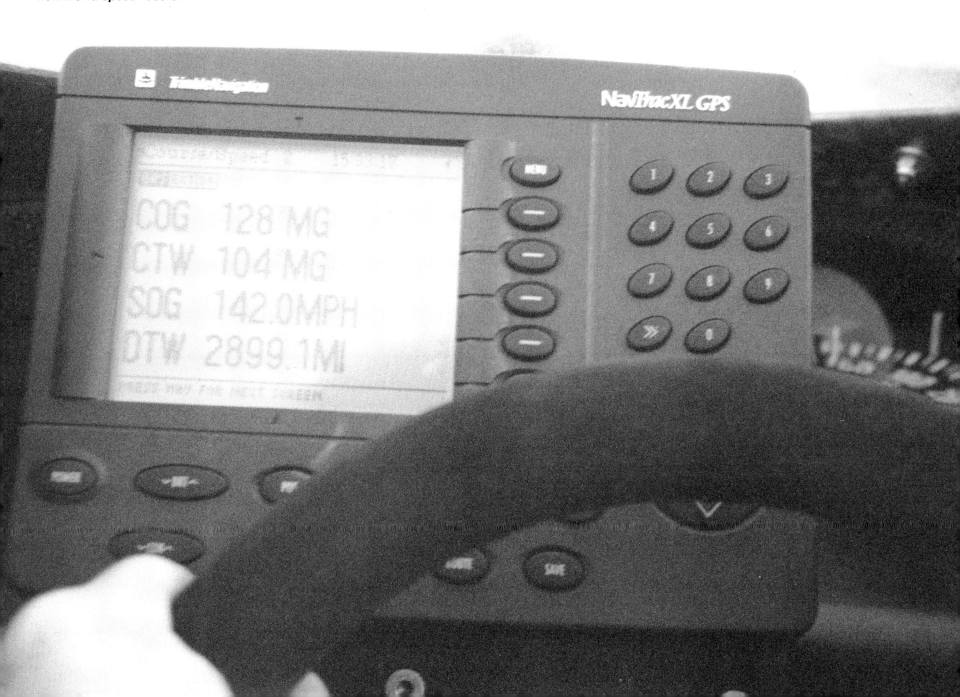

The NavTrac tells the story of the BP Valentino on its way to setting a new world speed record.

Hanging Up His Helmet

Andreas knew that retiring would be hard on him, but he didn't want to think about. Like Jann he spent the season avoiding any thought about retirement until it hit him while having dinner at the Ostend, Belgium Grand Prix.

The original Sunday race was held over an extra day when the rush of sea-going spectators ran out of control, making the course dangerous for both competitors and fans. Stopping the race mid-way, the organizers elected to reschedule for the next day, sending everyone into a flurry of activity; crew chiefs were off prepping the boat yet again, team members rushed to rework their travel plans, and publicity associates sent out a stack of press releases explaining the delay of the race.

That night at dinner the crew of *BP Valentino* sat in a quiet barbecue restaurant in Ostend. As smoke filled the air and everyone was excitedly talking about the second start of the race Andreas suddenly looked at his team and said, "Listen to all of you! Listen how excited you are! We didn't even finish the race today and everyone is so happy to try again you'd think we'd already won."

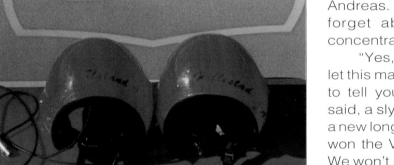

Andreas shook his head and cupped his chin in his hands. "I have to be out of my mind to think about leaving all this. What else is there left for us? What do we do? Go back to racing Class II or Class III? I tell you this...once you race the Grand Prix there's no turning back. There really is no turning back."

The happy group fell silent. Andreas turned, looking at his team and said. "I don't know how long I can stay away from this, but I have to. I just want to assure you that my passion will always be here..."

Jann smiled and said, "We know Andreas. What do you say we just forget about being sad and just concentrate on winning the race?"

"Yes, you're right. We shouldn't let this make us sad. Besides, I forgot to tell you all something," Andreas said, a sly smile on his face. "I bought a new long distance boat...the one that won the Venice to Monte Carlo race. We won't be on the Grand Prix, but we will run the Martini Series next year. It's only five races so it shouldn't affect my work too much"

As his happy voice trailed off into plans for the future the team looked at each other and grinned. Even if competing in less events, somehow Andreas had managed to make sure that the Ugland Team would keep on racing.

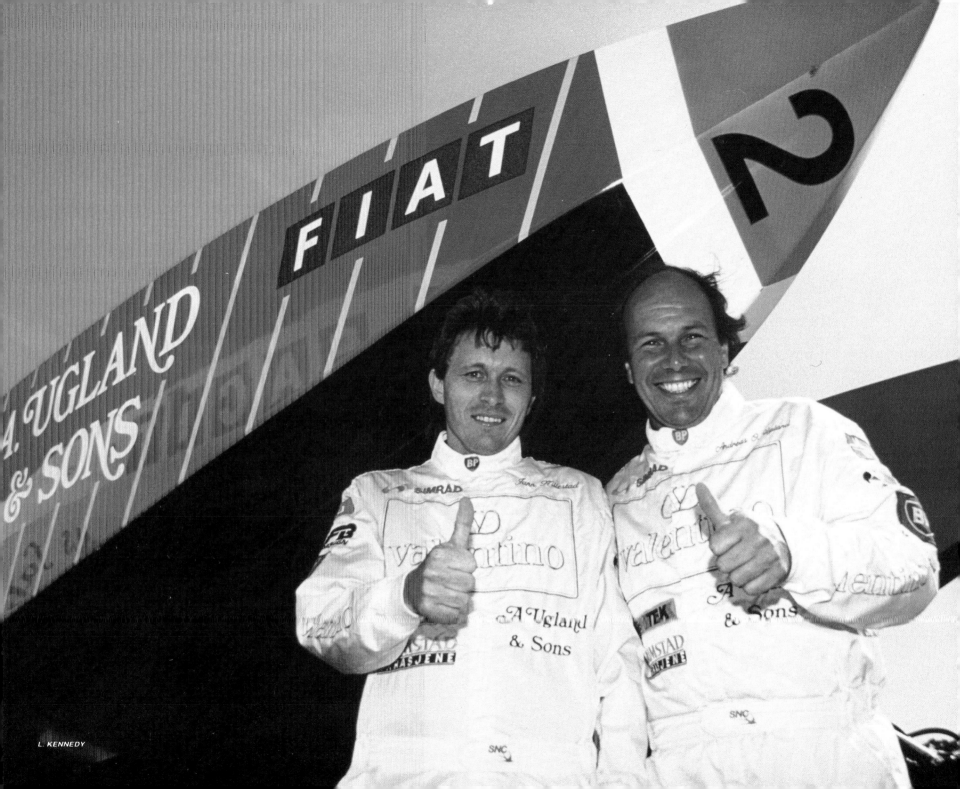